Emerging Infectious Diseases and Society

Also by Peter Washer

CLINICAL COMMUNICATION SKILLS

Emerging Infectious Diseases and Society

Peter Washer

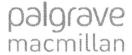

First published 2010 by
PALGRAVE MACMILLAN

Palgrave Macmillan in the UK is an imprint of Macmillan Publishers Limited, registered in England, company number 785998, of Houndmills, Basingstoke, Hampshire RG21 6XS.

Palgrave Macmillan in the US is a division of St Martin's Press LLC, 175 Fifth Avenue, New York, NY 10010.

Palgrave Macmillan is the global academic imprint of the above companies and has companies and representatives throughout the world.

Palgrave® and Macmillan® are registered trademarks in the United States, the United Kingdom, Europe and other countries.

ISBN-13: 978-0-230-22132-1 hardback

This book is printed on paper suitable for recycling and made from fully managed and sustained forest sources. Logging, pulping and manufacturing processes are expected to conform to the environmental regulations of the country of origin.

A catalogue record for this book is available from the British Library.

Library of Congress Cataloging-in-Publication Data
Washer, Peter.
    Emerging infectious diseases and society / Peter Washer.
        p.   cm.
    ISBN 978-0-230-22132-1 (hardback)
    1. Emerging infectious diseases—Popular works.   I. Title.
    RA643.W27 2010
    362.196'9—dc22   2010002717

Printed and bound in the United States of America

For Efisio

Contents

List of Figures

Preface

This book tells the story of the creation of a new medical category – emerging and re-emerging infectious diseases (EID) – and tracks the way that the central concepts behind this category have moved from the realms of science and public health to the realm of 'common sense'. In doing so, it describes how the idea that infectious diseases were 'conquered' and 'a thing of the past' has been replaced by the feeling that infectious diseases now threaten 'our' futures (in the developed world). In an attempt to provide a deeper sociocultural and political context to phenomenon of EID, the biomedical factors which have caused infectious diseases to 'emerge' are linked to the social and political processes underlying them. In short, this book unpacks what infectious diseases *mean* at this particular point in our history.

The subject matter cuts across several academic disciplines, including sociology, anthropology, psychology, geography, media studies, public health and the history of medicine. I hope that this may be of value to students and scholars in these various subjects and also that it will also be of interest to biomedical scientists, public health and healthcare professionals interested in a wider sociocultural perspective on contemporary infectious diseases. Not least, I hope that this book will be of interest to the general reader. In writing with such a wide audience in mind, I have tried not to assume any prior knowledge in any of the various fields covered.

Much of what is already written about EID describes them either in biomedical terms, or in terms of the history of medicine. Analyses of contemporary infectious diseases as sociocultural phenomena are less common. The one notable exception is HIV/AIDS, which a range of authors have elucidated in terms of the cultural impact of the epidemic. The meanings of other epidemics, such as Ebola, SARS and 'mad cow disease', have been analysed in similar ways by various social scientific studies. This book describes and builds on this work, and is indebted to it, but also applies the same level of analysis to the EID category, as a accumulation of all these various diseases.

EID have produced a plethora of fictionalised accounts and popular science books, many scholarly, some lurid. Yet despite the interest that the subject garners in the media, surprisingly the EID category itself has received relatively little analysis as a sociocultural and political phenomenon. This book addresses that gap by examining EID as a socially constructed category, with meanings and functions that go beyond and beneath the surface of the biomedical discourse. It aims to contextualise infectious diseases in terms of their social history, and also to examine how they have become increasingly politicised in the late modern, globalised world.

I would like to thank the following people for their help and encouragement while writing this book. Firstly, all my friends and family, who have given me so much support during the years while it has been in production, especially Rowan, who has been denied the company and attention of his father for too long. I owe a debt of gratitude to Olivia Middleton and Philippa Grand, my editors at Palgrave, who allowed me to extend deadline after deadline with patience and good grace; to Ali Glenny, for correcting my grammar; and to the library staff at St Mary's Hospital, Paddington – those unsung heroes of academia – who obliged me with a relentless supply of inter-library loans. My thanks also go to Brian Balmer, Ann Herring, Helene Joffe, Carol Pellowe, Stephen Smith and Jon Turney, and to my anonymous reviewers, who read earlier drafts and offered much-valued suggestions for improvement. Finally, I want to thank my partner Efisio, who has supported me morally and practically on this journey more than I could possibly repay, and to whom this book is dedicated.

Peter Washer

Introduction

Since the appearance of AIDS in the 1980s infectious diseases have made a resurgence, both medically and as a cultural and social phenomenon. The 1990s witnessed the creation of a new medical category – emerging or re-emerging infectious diseases (EID). This category has since become established in scientific discourse, and increasingly widely used in the mass media. Even if the term 'emerging infectious diseases' may be unfamiliar to many laypeople, the notion that infectious diseases are 'emerging or re-emerging' has to a certain extent become common sense. Some of the diseases that fall under the EID category are genuinely new, such as HIV/AIDS. Others are older diseases that are causing concern because of their reappearance when they had been apparently in decline, or because the bacteria and viruses that cause them are becoming increasing virulent or resistant to established treatments. This book will analyse the reasons behind this renewed interest in infectious disease from a biomedical perspective, but will also examine the sociocultural and political functions that infectious diseases serve in late modern society.

The opening chapter describes the creation of the new category, and will examine why there was a renewed interest and concern about infectious diseases in the 1990s. It will describe the characteristics of the modern world that are said to be causing infectious diseases to emerge or re-emerge. The authors of the new EID category used the newsworthiness of diseases such as AIDS and Ebola to attract attention, although they were equally or more concerned with developments such as the re-emergence of tuberculosis in the USA and the emergence of antibiotic-resistant strains of bacteria. The new category was disseminated though US government agencies, international bodies such as the World Health Organization and to the public through contact with journalists and popular science writers. In a process that will be familiar to philosophers and historians of science, the building of the new discipline involved publishing books and establishing journals dedicated to the subject, and later an infrastructure of academic posts and a conference circuit. The establishment of the EID paradigm proved extremely successful. It has become increasingly central to the way policy makers, the media and the general public conceptualise infectious disease.

The next chapter steps back to pose the question: Why did the authors of this new category feel it necessary to refocus attention onto infectious diseases in the early 1990s? It describes the reasons behind the optimism that infectious diseases had been 'conquered'. There *were* enormous gains in reducing illness and death from infectious diseases during the twentieth century, because of general improvements in public health, vaccination campaigns, and as a result of the introduction of antibiotics. This is particularly true in the developed world, but also in the developing world. Consequently, by the 1980s, medical research resources and public concern were focused on the so-called 'diseases of civilisation'. As epitomised in the epidemiological transitions theory, there was a widespread feeling that infectious diseases were a 'thing of the past', and that all countries, albeit on different time scales, were progressing towards a future where cardiovascular disease, cancer (and accidents) would overtake them as the main causes of death.

The appearance of AIDS in the early 1980s ended that optimism. AIDS was pivotal in changing the mood around infectious diseases, and in the birth of the EID category. In Chapter 3, the symbols and metaphors by which the public(s) collectively came to make sense of AIDS will be examined. It will describe the shifting conceptions of who was at risk and who was to blame for the new disease. AIDS shattered the hope that infectious diseases were conquered, or at least conquerable. The meanings attributed to AIDS marked a break with history in that it ended the widespread twentieth-century optimism that modern biomedicine could offer freedom from fear of infectious disease.

The factors that are said to lead to the emergence of infectious diseases are in many ways a list of the characteristics of late modernity: particularly (mis)use of technology, globalisation, increasing disparities of wealth and the mass migration associated with these developments. Chapter 4 breaks the forward thrust of the narrative by exploring various social theories around modernity, globalisation and risk and attempts to elucidate EID in terms of those theories. In particular, it will examine the way that migration has become increasingly 'securitised'. While immigrants have historically been blamed for the infections they are said to carry with them, the new discourse around migration also conceptualises them as posing a threat to 'our' way of life.

Chapter 5 describes the epidemics of infectious diseases that occurred after the establishment of the new EID category. In particular, it will examine how these epidemics were depicted and disseminated via the newly globalised media. This chapter examines the appearance of 'mad cow disease', Ebola, 'superbugs', 'bird flu' and SARS. Each of these infectious diseases were marked by a ratcheting up of the risk discourse, and a propensity to scapegoat and blame.

People in modern, technologically advanced societies like to think that their ideas about disease and contagion are based on 'scientific' principles such as their knowledge of germ theory. Yet the discourse around diseases like AIDS or SARS tended to be couched in the language of accusation, blame and religious fundamentalism. Connecting to patterns of blame from pre-modern eras, contemporary infectious diseases are often blamed either on 'dirty foreigners', 'promiscuous' gay men, 'prostitutes', 'junkies' and so on. These *othering* mechanisms serve to distance the threat that infectious diseases may pose to 'people like us'. *Others*, either 'foreigners' or marginalised groups in the host society, are blamed and stigmatised for infectious diseases. *Others* are at risk and to blame because they are dirty, eat disgusting food, have bizarre rituals or customs and have perverted or promiscuous sex.

A recurring motif in this blaming discourse relates to ideas about dirt and dirtiness, and this is enmeshed in related notions of morality and germs. Chapter 6 attempts to unravel the contemporary lay discourse about germs by tracing notions of dirt and contagion from their pre-bacteriological understandings, through early twentieth-century germ phobia to more recent understandings of the immune system. This detour will contextualise the sociocultural reaction to EID in terms of the reactions to historical epidemics such as cholera.

The EID worldview had become so established by the late 1990s that the ways of thinking it had engendered were transposed onto the entirely separate issue of terrorism. Concerns about the potential of terrorists using biological weapons against American civilian targets predate the 2001 anthrax letters attacks by at least a decade. Chapter 7 explores the issue of bioterrorism, and how the issue of US public health became increasingly 'securitised'. For public health officials, this alleged bioterror threat presented an opportunity to obtain badly needed resources. The alleged threat to America and American citizens from both EID and from potential bioterrorist attacks seemed to call for the same 'dual-use' response, namely an improved public infrastructure and tightened border controls. The meshing together of bioterrorism and EID also served the political agenda of the Republican hawks of President George W. Bush's administration.

Connected with the 'securitisation' of migration, EID have increasingly become to be portrayed as a threat to global security. The final chapter will examine how the apparently deteriorating condition of global public health has raised concerns, not primarily because of the suffering of the people affected, but because of the threat EID are said to pose to 'global' security. The EID discourse is often decontextualised from the lived experience of discrimination and inequality suffered by those people affected by them. The final discussion of the book is an attempt to provide an often-lacking political and economic context to EID. I hope that this book will provide a more nuanced understanding of the role of social injustice and unequal distribution of our world's resources in the 'emergence or re-emergence' of infectious diseases.

1
Factors in the Emergence of Infectious Diseases

In 1989, a new branch of medicine was born, one which would turn on its head previous scientific and lay thinking about infectious diseases and would mark an end to the optimism that had previously characterised the *conquest of infectious diseases*. This creation of this new category – 'emerging and re-emerging infectious diseases' – represents a tectonic shift in biomedical thinking and has became increasingly central to the way policy-makers, the media and the general public conceptualise infectious disease. Who were the authors of this new category? What were the concerns that prompted its creation and what were social and political forces that lay behind it?

On 1 May 1989, a conference was held in Washington DC, sponsored by the US National Institutes of Health (NIH) in cooperation with The Rockefeller University. The theme of the conference was *Emerging Viruses: The Evolution of Viruses and Viral Diseases*. The conference was chaired by Stephen Morse, Assistant Professor of Virology at the university. As a virologist, Morse's concern was with new viral illnesses, particularly human immunodeficiency virus (HIV), as well as with more exotic viral illnesses affecting humans, such as Ebola. Speakers also presented papers on new viral illnesses affecting animals, such as canine distemper and seal plague virus. The keynote speaker at that conference, and author of the first chapter in the subsequent book based on its proceedings (*Emerging Viruses* Morse, 1992b) was the Nobel Laureate molecular biologist Joshua Lederberg. One of the central themes of the conference was that new viral illnesses 'emerged' as an evolutionary response to human-made changes in the environments of viruses. A similar evolutionary strategy accounted for bacterial resistance to antibiotics, and Lederberg, in his address, coined the term 'emergent diseases' (Bud, 2006).

As a result of that conference, in 1991 the US Institute of Medicine (IOM) and the National Academy of Sciences convened a *Committee on Emerging Microbial Threats to Health*, chaired by Lederberg. The committee included experts in the fields of epidemiology, virology, biology, parasitology and infectious diseases. Their remit was to address not just viral, but *all* emerging microbial threats to the health of Americans. The term 'emerging or re-emerging infectious diseases' (EID) derives from the report of that committee, published the following year as *Emerging Infections: Microbial Threats to Health in the United States* (Lederberg et al., 1992). In the IOM report, EID are defined as:

> ...clinically distinct conditions whose incidence in humans has increased... Emergence may be due to the introduction of a new agent, to the recognition of an existing disease that has gone undetected, or to a change in the environment that provides an epidemiologic 'bridge'... Emergence, or more specifically, re-emergence, may also be used to describe the reappearance of a known disease after a decline in incidence. Although an infectious agent plays a role in any emerging infectious disease, other causative factors may be important as well. (Lederberg et al., 1992: 34)

Infectious diseases are usually classified according to the type of microbe (virus, bacteria etc) that causes them, but in the IOM report, the new category of EID was described in terms of an interconnected list of factors related to their 'emergence'. By encompassing the common factors that lie behind all these diverse diseases, the EID category aimed to contextualise infectious diseases in terms of the wider social forces which lead to their appearance and spread. These factors were:

- Human demographics and behaviour.
- Technology and industry.
- Economic development and land use.
- International travel and commerce.
- Microbial adaptation and change.
- Breakdown of public health measures.

What then were the concerns of this group of doctors, scientists and epidemiologists in the late 1980s that made them feel that infectious diseases were 'emerging' to threaten the health of Americans?

Human demographics and behaviour

The first factor, or more precisely set of factors, said to lead to the emergence of new infectious diseases were those relating to human demographics and human behaviour. In order for a disease to 'emerge', a novel infection, whatever its origin, has first to be introduced into a new host population, through which it subsequently spreads. That dissemination usually occurs as a result of human social behaviour. The ability of a pathogen (a disease-causing microbe) to be transmitted between people is largely related to the density of the population susceptible to it. One of the features of the modern world is its unprecedented population growth, and in particular the worldwide trend towards urbanisation. As growing numbers of people, particularly in the developing world, move from the countryside into overcrowded cities and high-density urban slums, the overcrowding and lack of basic sanitation and public health measures they encounter there puts them at risk of infectious diseases.

Dengue, for example, is a tropical disease of early childhood and is spread by mosquitoes. It is one of the most prevalent human viral diseases, with an estimated 50–100 million cases of dengue fever and dengue haemorrhagic fever each year globally. Dengue virus is short-lived in humans, and therefore sustains itself most successfully in densely populated areas. The number of dengue outbreaks had risen dramatically since the early 1980s, particularly in the Americas and in Southeast Asia. Furthermore, international commerce in recycled goods, for example in used tyres imported from Japan to the USA, had been shown to cause invasions of infected mosquitoes in several southern US states.

Population density and lack of basic sanitation also accounts for the resurgence of infections like cholera in the developing world, particularly when they strike people already weakened by poverty and malnutrition. For example, after a 50-year period when cholera seemed to be receding, a new cholera epidemic caused by the *El Tor* strain emerged in 1961 in Indonesia, and by the 1970s had spread through trade, tourism and religious pilgrimage routes to Asia, parts of Europe and Africa. The *El Tor* epidemic of cholera continues to this day, and in 1992 a new strain of cholera – *V. Cholerae* 0139 – emerged in Madras, India, and spread quickly through Asia (Singel & Lashley, 2009).

Growing populations are also forced to expand into territory previously uninhabited by humans, such as virgin forests, where they can disturb zoonotic (animal) reservoirs of infections. At the time of the IOM report the evidence was still circumstantial, but it was widely

believed that the HIV virus was related to similar simian immunodeficiency viruses (SIV) found in African monkeys. The hypothesis was
that the virus had 'jumped species' to humans as a result of African
hunting of primates for food – so-called 'bushmeat'. The HIV epidemic
then spread in Africa through the 1960s and 1970s, driven by major
social upheavals related to the end of colonial rule in Africa, particularly
the civil wars that followed independence in many countries (Hahn &
Shaw, 2000; Hillis, 2000). At the same time in the USA and other developed countries, HIV was spreading as a result of different changes in
human behaviour, particularly those following the sexual revolution of
the 1960s, and the growing use of intravenous drugs.

In the developed nations in the latter half of the twentieth century,
another demographic shift was occurring. Largely as a result of the
decline in deaths from infectious diseases, the population in most Western countries was ageing. Diseases that would have been fatal before the
1960s and 1970s, such as chronic renal failure, became treatable with
medical interventions such as renal dialysis, and a range of different cancers were increasingly treatable with advances in surgery, chemotherapy
and radiotherapy. This growing population of people either suffering
from chronic disease, cancer or old age resulted in a corresponding
increase in immunocompromised people more vulnerable to infectious
diseases.

Technology and industry

As well as a growing and increasingly crowded human population,
and changes in human behaviour, a second consequence of human
action related to emergence of new infections related to technology
and industry, such as medical technologies and new methods of food
production.

As the population in developed countries aged, the average age
of hospitalised inpatients increased. Subsequently, so did the incidence of nosocomial (hospital or health care acquired) infections from
indwelling venous catheters, venous access devices and other facilita-
tors of infections. By the 1980s there was growing evidence that the
increasing sophistication of medical technology and procedures were
also facilitating a range of nosocomial infections. For example, hepatitis following blood transfusions was increasingly common, particularly
after the introduction in the 1950s of surgical procedures such as open
heart surgery and kidney transplantation, which required large amounts
of transfused blood. In some hospitals where these procedures were

performed, as many as 50 per cent of patients became infected and many became seriously ill. In 1965 Baruch Blumberg discovered the so-called *Australia antigen* associated with the hepatitis B virus (HBV), and a blood test was later developed to identify those infected. Research in the USA, Europe, Africa and Asia starting in the 1970s showed that HBV was the major cause of primary liver cancer, one of the world's most common cancers (Blumberg, 1977).

A safe and effective vaccine for HBV was developed in 1980 and licensed in 1982. Although the HBV vaccine offered no benefit for those already affected, it protected 90 per cent of those vaccinated against infection. Later blood screening and vaccine programmes were introduced, although there was little media interest in any of these developments at the time (Blumberg, 1988). By the mid 1980s there was an enormous increase in sexually-transmitted HBV in Western countries, with 80 per cent of certain populations of gay men infected, and a chronic carrier rate of between six and ten per cent, although infections in gay men dropped dramatically after the adoption of safer-sex practices following the appearance of HIV (Muraskin, 1993).

After the two causative agents of the two transmissible forms of hepatitis, A and B, had been identified, it was clear that there was at least one more type of hepatitis, which at that time was called 'non-A non-B hepatitis'. This was responsible for disease in a large number of transfusion recipients and injecting drug users. This was later found to be a third virus, named hepatitis C virus (HCV), which was isolated in 1989. HCV was later recognised to be the leading cause of chronic liver disease and liver cancer (Davey, 2002). HCV is less infectious than HBV, but developing a vaccine against it has not proved possible because HCV mutates so rapidly.

As well as advances in medical technology, another set of technological factors facilitating the emergence of new infectious diseases related to changes in the way food was produced, processed and handled. Increasing population and urbanisation inevitably leads to the need for food to be mass produced, and then stored, transported and distributed. In the last 100 years, large-scale food processing and distribution has been developed to meet this need. Modern food production followed the mechanisation of farms and subsequent urbanisation of the rural population; together with the simultaneous advent of railroads, which made possible first shipping the harvest to food manufacturers and then shipping packaged food on to the urban consumer (Urquhart & Heilmann, 1984). Modern food production is also increasingly globalised, with consumers in developed nations demanding foods once considered exotic or demanding out-of-season foods all year round (Chavers et al., 2002).

In the past, food poisoning outbreaks would usually follow an event such as a family picnic or a wedding reception, and were acute and local with a large number of people affected. Thus the outbreaks were immediately apparent to medical and public health authorities, and were usually traced to a food handling error in a small kitchen that occurred shortly before consumption. However, because of changes in the way food is produced and distributed, a new kind of pattern of food poisoning has appeared, often with widespread outbreaks in many geographical locations as a result of low-level contamination of a widely distributed commercial food product. This new type of outbreak would often be detected only because of a chance concentration of cases in one location, and would often be a result of contamination somewhere in the industrial chain of food production (Tauxe, 1997).

Escherichia coli is a microbe normally found in the gut of humans and animals. In 1982, a new and deadly strain – *E. Coli* O157: H7 – was first identified in the USA. *E. Coli* O157: H7 produces toxins similar to those produced by dysentery-causing *Shigella dysenteriae*. For most people this will result in severe diarrhoea that usually subsides after a week. However in about six per cent of patients, and particularly in children and the elderly, it is associated with a post-diarrhoeal haemolytic uremic syndrome (HUS), and can lead to acute renal failure. About a quarter of those with HUS develop neurological symptoms such as seizures; 5 per cent have serious long-term consequences such as end-stage renal disease or permanent neurological injury; and 3 per cent die (Boyce et al., 1996).

Inference from data on the incidence of HUS suggests that *E. Coli* O157: H7 has probably been present and increasing slowly since 1955, when HUS was first described (Boyce et al., 1996), although much of the apparent increase in outbreaks can be accounted for by increased laboratory screening. Unlike many EID, *E. Coli* O157: H7 appears to be mainly a disease of industrialised countries, and cases have been most commonly reported from Canada and the USA (Tartasky, 2002). The majority of outbreaks have been as a result of foods of a bovine origin, and its recent emergence can probably be accounted for by changes in rearing, slaughtering and processing cattle. In addition, per capita consumption of ground (minced) beef in the USA had risen by 23 per cent between 1970 and 1993 (Boyce et al., 1996). *E Coli* O157:H7 has been responsible for large food-borne outbreaks in the USA, Europe and Japan and was the cause of over 600 cases of food poisoning from the 'Jack-in-a-Box' fast food restaurants in Washington State in 1992, as a result of which 45 people developed HUS and three toddlers died (Levy & Fischetti, 2003).

By the end of 1987, bovine spongiform encephalopathy (BSE) – so-called 'mad cow disease' – had been reported in cattle herds in all the mainland regions of the UK, and the numbers of herds reported to have been affected by it was rising rapidly. The 1989 report of the British government-commissioned Southwood Committee argued that BSE was a form of scrapie, a disease of sheep that did not cause disease in humans. The report argued that the jump between sheep and cows had been caused by cows being fed the processed carcasses of scrapie-infected sheep. As people had eaten scrapie-infected sheep for many years and had not become infected, the committee argued that cattle infected with BSE were also likely to prove a 'dead end host' and that the infection was unlikely to have any implications for human health. The report predicted that the disease would disappear in cows some time after 1996 (Lacey, 1994). However, even at the time of the publication of the IOM report in 1992, many people were arguing that there was a possibility that BSE could similarly 'jump species' from cows and could infect humans. As discussed in Chapter 5, it was only later, in 1996, that the link between so-called 'mad cow disease' and the human form of the disease was confirmed.

Economic development and land use

About three-quarters of EID, particularly those caused by viruses, are not newly evolved pathogens, but are zoonotic, meaning that they are already existing agents whose common natural reservoirs are in animals, most often rodents (Morse, 1992a; Taylor et al., 2001). Thus, the IOM report highlighted a further set of factors that increased the potential for diseases to 'emerge' that related to economic development and changes to land use, particularly those that put humans at risk of contracting zoonotic diseases.

Paradoxically, while deforestation can lead to the emergence of infectious diseases, *reforestation* can also provide increased opportunities for zoonotic infections to emerge. This happened in 1975 in Old Lyme, Connecticut, when a cluster of about a dozen children were found to be suffering from long bouts of fever and aching joints, and were initially diagnosed with juvenile rheumatoid arthritis. Many parents recalled the children having been bitten by a tick and then having developed a rash when the illness started. In 1981 the bacterium *Borrelia burgdorferi* was identified as the cause, and the subsequent disease came to be known as Lyme disease. Lyme disease is not strictly speaking new, but is novel as an epidemic, caused by changes to the environment, namely reforestation of deforested areas causing an increase in the population of deer and the deer tick, which is the organism that carries bacterium from one host to another (the vector). As suburban development moved closer to reforested areas, people began to live in closer proximity to deer.

Another change in land use that can lead to emergence of EID relates to the stimulation of growth in mosquito populations by dam building. For example, following dam construction on the Senegal River, a Rift Valley fever epidemic occurred for the first time in Mauritania, and another in Egypt followed the opening of the Aswan dam (Hui, 2006).

Another development that alarmed the authors of the IOM report was the emergence of haemorrhagic fevers in the USA in the years preceding the report. There are three 'classic' haemorrhagic fevers: yellow fever (see Chapter 2) and dengue, which are transmitted by mosquitoes, and hanta virus, which is a natural infection of the field mouse and can cause a range of illnesses including haemorrhagic fever with renal syndrome (HFRS).

Human disease due to hantaviral infections first came to the attention of Western medicine during the Korean War, when a 'new' disease – Korean haemorrhagic fever – was observed amongst United Nations forces. Over 2,000 US troops were infected and many fatalities occurred. Haemorrhagic fevers had been well known in many parts of Asia and Northern Europe for many years, but had always been a rare disease appearing in sparsely populated rural areas. It was not until the isolation of Hantaan virus in 1976 that a specific virus could be associated with the disease, named after the Hantaan River, near the epidemic centre in Korea (LeDuc et al., 1993).

Hantaan virus is probably a virus that has coevolved with its rodent host over many years but the virus 'emerged' as a result of expanded rice production, which created new opportunities for human contact with infected rodents during rice harvests. In the 1980s, the World Health Organization (WHO) endorsed the term 'haemorrhagic fever with renal syndrome' (HFRS) as a generic term to cover all hantaviral disease. The virus accounts for over 100,000 cases of disease in China alone, and there are related forms found in other parts of the world: Puumala virus found in Scandinavia and Northern Europe, which causes a less severe form of HFRS, and Porogia virus, found in the Balkan Region, which causes a very severe form of HFRS (LeDuc et al., 1993).

In 1993 there was an outbreak of Hantavirus pulmonary syndrome (HPS) amongst 17 Navajo people in New Mexico, caused by what became known as the Sin Nombre Virus, which caused 14 deaths, mostly amongst previously healthy young people (Groom & Cheek, 2002). Similarly, in South America, Argentine hemorrhagic fever, another rodent infection caused by Junin virus, emerged as a result of conversion of grassland to maize cultivation (Morse, 1995). The problem of deforestation and development, and expanding agriculture into forests continues to create similar opportunities for zoonotic infections to jump into humans. In Malaysia in 1998, for example, there was an outbreak of the Nipah virus as a result of deforestation (Hui, 2006).

Although not related to human activity, global changes in climate, such as high rainfall during *El Niño*, can also lead to an increase in mosquito-borne diseases. At the time of the publication of the IOM report in 1992, global warming was 'still a controversial issue', but the report nevertheless predicted that global warming could trigger mosquito-based infections in novel geographical locations.

International travel and commerce

A further set of factors said to lead to the emergence of infectious diseases related to international travel and commerce. Travel by humans, and the animal vectors such as rats that humans carry with them, has been a pathway for disseminating infectious diseases throughout history. However, it is the volume, speed and reach of modern travel that is unprecedented. This massive movement of animals, humans and goods allows for mixing diverse genetic pools of microbes, both of humans and animals, at rates and in combinations previously unknown (Wilson, 1995).

International air travel had led to a number of cases of 'exotic' diseases in developed nations. For example, there had been occasional reports of Lassa fever in the 1980s in the USA and Europe in people who were infected in Africa, where it is endemic (always present) in nations such as Guinea, Sierra Leone and Nigeria. Lassa virus is a member of the family of viruses known as *Arenaviridae* or arenaviruses, which includes Junin, Machupo, and Guanarito viruses. The animal reservoir of arenaviruses is in rodents, and transmission to humans occurs through contact with rodent droppings. Lassa fever had been described in the 1950s in native populations of West Africa but first came to world attention in 1969, when two missionary nurses in Jos, Nigeria, contracted a mysterious fever while caring for patients in a mission hospital (Ellis & Lashley, 2002).

As well as the potential of microbes to travel in the bodies of infected humans, they also travelled in the bodies of animals transported around the world for scientific experiments, for the pet trade and for food. Vectors of diseases, such as mosquitoes, have also survived in the wheel bays of international airplane flights. In 1967 there was a lethal outbreak of a haemorrhagic fever in Marburg and Frankfurt, Germany, and in Belgrade in the former Yugoslavia. The outbreak was traced to a shipment of vervet or African green monkeys imported from Uganda, and the cause was named *Marburg virus*.

Marburg remained an obscure medical curiosity until 1976, when there were two epidemics of haemorrhagic fever in small rural African communities. In N'zara, a town in Southern Sudan close to the border of Zaire (now Congo), 284 people contracted the disease and 151 (53 per cent) died. This outbreak, apparently centred on a local cotton factory, seems to have been the source for another outbreak in the Bumba Zone in Zaire. The epidemic was marked by a high transmission rate amongst friends, family and medical staff who had had prolonged and close contact with the sick, although the virus was apparently transmitted via contact with infected blood, rather than by an airborne route. In one local hospital, the doctor-in-charge and 61 members of the 154 nursing staff developed the disease, and 33 died, with a further eight deaths amongst cleaners and ancillary staff (Deng et al., 1978).

Isolation of viruses from both epidemics led to the discovery of the *Ebola* virus, named after a local river. Ebola is presumed to have an animal reservoir and it is known to affect gorillas and chimpanzees. Indeed, Ebola threatens their survival in their last stronghold in Equatorial Africa, where declines of more than 50 per cent in the population of gorillas and chimpanzees between 1983 and 2000 are partly blamed on the disease (Kuiken et al., 2003).

Both Marburg and Ebola were found to be members of a new family of viruses, the *Filoviridae* or filoviruses. After the 1976 epidemics, filoviruses once again largely disappeared from mainstream medical interest, although there continued to be isolated human cases and small outbreaks. Although filoviruses were capable of causing human disease with high mortality and person-to-person spread, they were sufficiently rare not to present a major health threat.

That perception changed in 1989, when an outbreak of an Ebola-like epidemic was reported to be spreading amongst macaque monkeys imported from the Philippines into a US quarantine facility at Reston, Virginia. One of the animal technicians at Reston then developed a febrile illness, leading to a major incident alert. He later proved *not* to have Ebola, and in the event there were no human cases, as the strain turned out to be harmless to humans (Peters et al., 1993). The Ebola outbreak at Reston was later to be the subject of a popular science book *The Hot Zone* (Preston, 1995), which inspired the Hollywood film *Outbreak* a year later.

Microbial adaptation and change

A further set of factors causing the emergence of new infectious diseases highlighted in the IOM report related to evolutionary changes in microbes themselves. This can occur either through normal variation of the microbe, particularly those viruses that have a high rate of mutation, or through selective evolutionary pressure caused by the use of antimalarials and antibiotics, leading to new strains of antibiotic-resistant microbes.

Many EID are caused by RNA viruses that have high mutation rates, leading to rapid evolution and environmental adaptability. HIV, for example, evolves so quickly that the infection within a single person quickly becomes a quasi-species consisting of thousands of evolutionary variants (Palumbi, 2001a). As described above, HCV also mutates so quickly that it has proven impossible to develop a vaccine against it. Another virus with a high mutation rate is influenza, and different influenza strains, such as those from birds and pigs can reassort to produce a new virus that can infect humans.

Human activity has also led to evolutionary changes in microbes through the use of antimalarials. Starting in 1958, the UN Global Malaria Eradication Program was backed by US$110 million from the US Congress. Around the world, the WHO spread 400,000 tons of the pesticide dichlorodiphenyltrichloroethane (DDT), which is credited with saving 15 to 25 million lives. At first DDT succeeded, so that for example in Sri Lanka cases of malaria fell from one million in 1955 to less than two dozen in 1961. However, in that same year it was found that both the mosquito vectors and the *Plasmodium* pathogen they carried had evolved resistance to DDT, and the effort to eradicate malaria eventually failed. Environmentally, DDT was a disaster and caused widespread deaths of marine, bird and insect life. Rachael Carson's classic book *Silent Spring* (Carson, 1962) brought the damage caused by DDT to the public's consciousness. By 1972, having spent US$1 billion on malaria eradication, the WHO declared the programme dead, leaving poor countries with new strains of malaria and mosquitoes that are very hard to kill. By 1990, over 500 species of mosquito had evolved resistance to DDT (Palumbi, 2001b; Palumbi, 2001a).

In terms of bacterial mutations, the main reason for the rise in nosocomial infections seen by the 1980s was the explosion in the use of antibiotics. For example, in 1962, US hospitals purchased US$94 million worth of antibiotics, but by 1971 this figure had risen to US$218 million and by 1991 to US$3 billion (Fisher 1994). By the 1980s there were three particular strains of antibiotic-resistant infections that were raising particular alarm – meticillin-resistant *Staphylococcus aureus* (MRSA), vancomycin-resistant *Enterococci* (VRE), and multi-drug-resistant tuberculosis (MDR-TB).

Staphylococcus aureus is often found on the skin of healthy people, where it usually causes no problems. It can cause anything from skin rashes to pneumonia, particularly when people are immunocompromised due to other illnesses. Before the introduction of antibiotics in the 1940s, staphylococci were responsible for most hospital infections, primarily pneumonias, and after the introduction of penicillin in the 1940s these became well controlled. However, by the 1950s, penicillin-resistant strains of staphylococci had emerged and a dramatic resurgence of infections was seen in hospitals.

In the 1960s, new antibiotics – meticillin and cephalosporin – were introduced. These subdued penicillin-resistant staphylococci for a while, but by the end of the 1960s strains of MRSA had appeared in New York and parts of Canada, Europe and Africa. In the late 1960s and 1970s, MRSA started to disappear from the UK, Denmark, Australia and several other countries. The reason for this disappearance is unclear, but again for reasons that remain uncertain, in the 1980s, new strains emerged again in Australia, the USA and Eire, and then in the UK and other countries (Wellcome Witnesses to Twentieth Century Medicine, 2000). In 1987, another new antibiotic – ciprofloxacin – was introduced, although soon MRSA also became resistant to it. By 1990, the spread of MRSA around the world had reached critical levels.

The only antibiotic that could be used against MRSA was vancomycin. Developed in the 1950s, vancomycin had remained largely unused owing to its toxicity, with side-effects that included kidney damage and hearing loss, and because of its poor absorbability, which meant that it had to be administered intravenously. It was also expensive: when the

FDA licensed it in 1958 it cost US$100 a day per patient. When meticillin was released in 1960, vancomycin was all but forgotten, but by the 1980s the toxicity of vancomycin became less significant in light of it being the only drug that consistently worked against MRSA (Shnayerson & Plotkin, 2002).

Enterococci are another important cause of nosocomial infections, and the antibiotic therapy of choice for enterococcal infections was ampicillin. However, strains of Enterococci emerged in the 1980s in the USA that were resistant to ampicillin. As well as increased use of vancomycin to treat MRSA in the late 1980s, there was an increased use of vancomycin to treat antibiotic-associated diarrhoea and colitis due to *Clostridium difficile* (Rice, 2001).

By 1986 the inevitable had happened, and there were reports of enterococcal infections that were resistant to vancomycin. By the early 1990s, VRE was spreading in hospitals through both person-to-person spread and through selective antibiotic pressure, particularly in those patients who had prolonged stays in hospital, who had been in intensive care units, and who had had organ transplants and cancers such as leukaemia (Rice, 2001). By 1993 VRE had become epidemic in many hospitals on both sides of the Atlantic and was all but untreatable, with mortality rates of more than 40 per cent. In the USA and elsewhere, both MRSA and VRE spread from the intensive care units of large teaching hospitals, outwards to other wards, then to other hospitals and finally to long-term care facilities. While MRSA had taken 15 years to spread across the USA (and remained susceptible to vancomycin), VRE took just five years to spread, and was of course vancomycin-resistant (Shnayerson & Plotkin, 2002).

In Europe, the appearance of VRE may also be related to the use of a vancomycin-like antibiotic – avoparcin – having been added to animal feed. Such use accounts for approximately half of all the antibiotics manufactured (Stokes, 2002). Adding antibiotics to animal feed was initially done to prevent bacterial pathogens common in intensive farming, but was then added to enhance the animals' growth rate. Animals fed on avoparcin are more likely to yield VRE than animals from farms where it is not used (Khardori, 2002). Although the use of avoparcin in animal feed was banned in the European Union in 1997, VRE is present in up to 10 per cent of the human population in Europe as a result of its use (Kaufmann, 2009). Food products contaminated with VRE and VRE-colonised animals may thus serve as a reservoir from which non-hospitalised patients can acquire VRE. Since the 1990s there have been fears that MRSA is also developing resistance to vancomycin, and there have already been cases of MRSA which are at least partially resistant to it.

As well as concerns about MRSA and VRE, another important driver behind the creation of the new EID category was the epidemic of tuberculosis (TB) that struck New York and several other major US inner cities in the late 1980s and early 1990s. Following the introduction of effective medical treatments for TB in the 1950s, by the 1970s TB had all but disappeared across the USA. As a result, between 1965 and 1989 TB control measures were dismantled. In 1972 TB project grants were replaced by general federal grants, and local governments began to shift funds elsewhere. Compared to research into cancer and heart disease, TB control and prevention lacked prestige in the medical world, and by 1979 the number of new research grants for the disease had dropped significantly (Smith-Nonini, 2004).

Reflecting the national picture, TB had declined in New York City (NYC), so that by 1968 the mayor had convened a Task Force to plan its elimination from the remaining small pockets, envisioning a TB free city. The Task Force recommended closing beds reserved for TB patients and relying on anti-TB drugs, so in the early 1970s, 13 of New York's 21 TB clinics were closed. In the mid-1970s the city's fiscal crisis led to health department staffing being cut by a quarter, which also badly affected TB control. In 1975–6 the incidence of TB rose two years in a row, followed by an extremely rapid decline for two years. After 1978, the incidence of TB in NYC again rose gradually each year. This was widely blamed in the medical literature on patients' failings – 'non-compliance' – rather than on structural causes such as poverty or the functioning of the health services. The incidence of TB in NYC continued to rise, following a classic upward epidemic curve, until it peaked in 1992. Eventually, people from nearly every ethnicity, class and age eventually became infected – only the very wealthiest most economically diverse neighbourhoods escaped the epidemic (Wallace & Wallace, 2003).

From 1985 onwards, there was also a progressive rise in new TB cases across the USA, yet from 1981 to 1987 the Reagan administration opposed a Federal programme against TB. In 1989 the increase in TB incidence in the USA was 4 per cent on the previous year, and by 1990 there was a 9.4 per cent jump, with over 25,000 Americans contracting TB. In Britain, TB had also been increasing since 1987, and by 1991 there were 1,794 cases in London, giving it one of the largest TB burdens of any city in the developed world. In 1992, the WHO warned that TB was rising in the industrialised world, naming as affected ten countries: Switzerland, Denmark, the Netherlands, Sweden, Norway, Austria, Ireland, Finland, Italy and the UK (Ryan, 1992).

The resurgence of TB in developed nations in the 1990s was particularly related to the AIDS epidemic. When people are co-infected with both HIV and TB there is a synergy that leads to HIV triggering latent TB infections, as well as TB having the capacity to activate HIV infection, causing it to lead to AIDS more rapidly, sometimes within only months of the host becoming infected with HIV. During a 1990 TB meeting of the WHO, Africa was described as 'lost', meaning that there was no way of dealing with the problems caused by co-infection with HIV and TB there. The description was not questioned by anyone at the meeting (Stanford & Grange, 1991).

By 1991, as TB had reached epidemic levels in NYC, the media also began to report that a drug-resistant strain of TB was causing deaths in New York's prisons. By then, multi-drug-resistant tuberculosis (MDR-TB) was already present in 13 states of the USA and in NYC (Reichman & Tanne, 2002). The cost to NYC of dealing with MDR-TB ran into millions of dollars and MDR-TB served as a catalyst, forcing restructuring of the health bureaucracy and new funding to TB programmes. Yet even after an announcement in 1990 by the NYC authorities of a dramatic rise in TB incidence, the George Bush Snr. administration cut the Center for Disease Control's TB control budget from US$36 to US$8 million (Smith-Nonini, 2004).

Breakdown in public health measures

The final factor described in the IOM report as being responsible for the emergence of infectious diseases was the dismantling and breakdown in public health measures.

Partly as a result of the triumphalism surrounding infectious diseases, the US Communicable Disease Center, the main US resource for tackling infectious disease, had changed its name in the 1970s to the Center for Disease Control (CDC), reflecting a new broader mission that included non-infectious diseases. In 1980, it became the Center for Disease Control and Prevention, reflecting its reorientation towards lifestyle and environmental issues. At the same time, on a Federal level, in 1981 the newly elected President Reagan called for a cut of 25 per cent in authorisations for health programmes, including all those implemented through the CDC and NIH. Throughout the 1980s, the Republican administrations maintained pressure to constrain budget requests (Smith-Nonini, 2004), and the visibility and emphasis on infectious diseases generally decreased as the Center established divisions for Chronic Disease Prevention and Health Promotion in 1989 and for Injury Control and Prevention in 1992 (Berkelman & Freeman, 2004).

Together with the re-emergence of TB, this shifting of focus and funding away from public health measures led to the appearance of several water-borne and food-borne infections in the USA. One of these newly identified pathogens was *Cryptosporidium*. Cryptosporidiosis had only been recognised as an infection in humans since 1967. In most people cryptosporidiosis causes self-limiting diarrhoea; however, the elderly, people with HIV and cancer, or those on immunosuppressive treatments, were more vulnerable, and they were more likely to have serious consequences when they contracted the infection (Hewitt & Schmid, 2002).

Another newly identified food-borne pathogen was *Cyclosporidium*, which had first been described as causing severe diarrhoea in humans in 1979. Identification of cyclospora began to be made more often after acid-fast staining was modified in the mid-1980s, facilitating its detection. Before that, some cases of diarrhoea caused by cyclospora would have been inaccurately diagnosed. In the late 1980s, cyclospora caused many cases of diarrheal illness in travellers returning to the USA from Haiti and Mexico (Lashley, 2002).

One final consequence of the breakdown in public health measures that had led to the resurgence of infections was under-vaccination against common diseases. In developed countries, a large number of diseases that only a generation or two previously had caused serious disease in children were, in effect, eradicated through widespread vaccination programmes. Measles, mumps, rubella (German measles), pertussis (whooping cough) and diphtheria had all but disappeared in developed countries. However, the combination of underfunded public health programmes, parental refusal to vaccinate and several scares about the safety of vaccines had led to declining rates of vaccinations, and inevitably the incidence many of these diseases rose.

The success of EID

The authors of the IOM report set out to refocus the attention of the scientific community, of (American) politicians and of the public onto the threat that infectious diseases continued to pose (to Americans). Like ripples in a pond, this new worldview – that infectious diseases were not a thing of the past, but were 'emerging or re-emerging' – spread out from the IOM report, to the CDC, to international organisations and into the consciousness of the public(s) across the world.

In 1994, the CDC responded to the IOM report with its own strategy document: *Addressing Emerging Infectious Disease Threats: A prevention strategy for the United States* (CDC, 1994), proposing improvements in infectious disease surveillance, applied research, prevention and control and infrastructure – this strategy was revised in 1998 (CDC, 1998). In 1995, the US National Science and Technology Council's Committee on International Science, Engineering and Technology (CISET) also published a report, *Global Microbial Threats in the 1990s*, which further recommended that the USA play a stronger role in global efforts to control infectious disease (National Science and Technology Council, 1995).

Also in 1995, the New York Academy of Medicine and the New York State Health Department convened a conference entitled *Emerging Infectious Diseases: Meeting the Challenge*. At the IOM's 25th anniversary annual meeting in October that year, where Joshua Lederberg was one of the featured speakers, they again focused on EID and devoted a major part of their scientific programme to the topic. 1995 also saw the CDC launch a new peer-reviewed quarterly journal, *Emerging Infectious Diseases*, which unlike most scientific journals that at that time required a subscription, was made freely available via the Internet. On the basis of the CISET report, President Clinton issued a Presidential Decision Directive in June 1996 establishing a national policy to address the threat of EID through improved domestic and international surveillance, prevention, and response measures. In the same year, 36 medical journals in 20 countries joined forces to focus attention on the subject of EID (Dismukes, 1996).

As well as successfully establishing the EID brand within the scientific and biomedical communities, National Center for Infectious Diseases (NCID) scientists were trained to work with the media and made special efforts to communicate with news reporters and science writers, responding to press inquiries more fully than had been their usual practice and encouraging journalists' interest. NCID scientists took steps to keep the writers Richard Preston and Laurie Garrett informed of the government's plans, knowing that both were speaking publicly on the issue of EID and were openly supportive in the media of the CDC's efforts. Garrett released her book *The Coming Plague* (Garrett, 1995) and Preston released *The Hot Zone* (Preston, 1995) soon after the publication of the IOM report.

The wrapper for marketing the concept to the lay public and politicians was adopted from scientific discussions about 'emerging' and 're-emerging' infections. A typical requirement for political marketability is the creation of the perception that what needs

action – and money – is both new and very important ... By grouping
the long list of disease-causing agents under one banner, 'the problem' to be addressed grew from a series of single diseases to a more
imposing aggregation imbued with newness. (Berkelman & Freeman,
2004: 369–70)

The IOM report thus heralded the start of a campaign that historians of
science recognise as the early stages of discipline-building, with repeated
rounds of conferences, a new journal and related papers published in
established journals, media-savvy scientists talking directly to journalists and science writers, and the issuing of press releases, all of which
became media events in their own right (King, 2004). Journalists were
thus able to characterise individual outbreaks of often rare or distant
infectious diseases as incidents of global significance. By aggregating a
range of diverse infectious diseases with different causes (viral, bacterial
etc), as well as different origins, severity and clinical consequences, the
authors of the EID category were able to focus attention on the long-
neglected issue of infectious diseases and public health. They presented
to the public and to politicians a frightening new threat that deserved
decisive political action and massive new streams of funding.

The new conceptual framework that the EID category represented
was promoted to international organisations like the WHO, which
established a 'Division of Emerging and Other Communicable Diseases
Surveillance and Control', making the issue a central part of its global
strategy (King, 2002). New funding streams from previously contracting
US Federal government sources were tapped by exploiting the political
and news profile of infectious diseases.

Within a few years, there was widespread acceptance of the new EID
framework from both US government agencies and international health
organisations. If the primary aim of the authors of the EID concept was
to raise awareness of the issue, the secondary aim was to attract funding
to infectious disease research and to the neglected public health infrastructure, both within America and outside its borders, at least to those
diseases that posed a threat to Americans. Total funding for EID to the
National Institute for Allergy and Infectious Diseases (NIAID), just one
of the NIH, increased from US$47 million in 1994 to more than US$1.7
billion by 2005. The CDC budget for EID, independent of monies for
control of other infectious diseases, had similarly grown to more than
US$125 million by 2008 (Alcabes, 2009).

The IOM report thus marks the 'emergence' of a new strand of
biomedical discourse, a new way of representing reality. In the years

since its conception, that new biomedical discipline has become well established. Prestigious universities now appoint professors of Emerging Infectious Diseases. A growing literature of books and journals, as well as an international conference circuit, are also dedicated to the subject.

However, the concerns about modern world leading to the re-emergence of infectious diseases contained within the EID world-view stretch far wider than the rarefied world of science. In parallel to the discipline-building around EID within the scientific and biomedical community, there has been an enormously increased interest in infectious diseases at a societal level. Numerous popular science books, some scholarly, others more lurid, have conveyed the apparent threat of EID to a wider public. Through these popular science books, and especially through the mass media news reportage, the concept of EID has passed from the sphere of scientific conferences and journals to the domain of lay knowledge or common sense.

The various ways in which EID are put to work in diverse contemporary sociocultural and political debates will thus form the subject of the rest of this book. First though, it will be necessary to take a step backwards and to reflect on why the original authors of the EID category felt it was necessary to draw attention to infectious diseases in the late 1980s. The next chapter will discuss why, by the late 1970s, in the consciousness of the medical and scientific establishment as well as the public, infectious diseases had come to be thought of as a 'thing of the past'.

2
The Conquest of Infectious Disease

The creation of the new emerging infectious diseases classification marked a definitive break with the optimism that had surrounded thinking about infectious diseases. By the late 1970s, a widely held belief had formed, in both scientific and in lay thinking, that infectious diseases were a thing of the past. As the EID worldview became popularised through the 1990s, that optimism was completely turned around, so that infectious diseases became thought of as new risks that threaten 'our' futures (in the developed world). Was the optimism that infectious diseases had been conquered justified? Did infectious diseases ever go away, or was the impression that they had simply an element in a wider faith that science would continually improve both the quality of life and longevity? What was the historical background to the gains that were made against infectious diseases?

Epidemiological transitions

Omran (1971) first proposed the theory of 'epidemiological transitions' in the early 1970s. On the basis of evidence of mortality patterns, this theory distinguishes three stages of epidemiological transition:

1. The first transition occurred after the change from hunter-gathering to agriculture about 10,000 years ago. This led to a long 'age of pestilence and famine', in which mortality was high and fluctuating, and average life expectancy was between 20 and 40 years. Some

commentators (see for example Weiss & McMichael, 2004) have argued that contained within this transition there were other transitions, the first in Classical times when Eurasian civilisations came into contact with different pools of infections, and the next when Europeans colonised the New World from around 1500 onwards, giving indigenous peoples Old World diseases such as measles and smallpox.

2. The theory holds that the next epidemiological transition occurs in Western Europe in the eighteenth and nineteenth centuries, largely in the wake of public health measures and improved nutrition, and later through advances in medicine. Epidemics of infectious diseases begin to decline in frequency and magnitude, resulting in the average life expectancy increasing steadily from about 30 to about 55 (Armelagos et al., 2005).

3. By the 1970s, so the epidemiological transitions theory proposed, most Western countries were in the beginning phase of a slow rise in degenerative and human-made diseases caused by radiation injury, accidents, occupational hazards and carcinogens. Mortality rates among younger people were continuing to decline and eventually would stabilise until life expectancy exceeds 70. In developing countries, high mortality (from infectious diseases) continued well into the twentieth century, but by the 1970s, so the theory proposed, a similar transition was also occurring there. In developing countries, however, this transition was independent of the socioeconomic level of the country, and was initiated by medical progress, organised health care, and disease control programmes that were usually internationally assisted and financed. From the perspective of the 1970s, the crucial factor in population growth was fertility rather than mortality from infectious diseases (Omran, 1983).

The age of pestilence and famine

Evidence from before the shift to an agricultural subsistence economy about 10,000 years ago, and evidence gained from existing hunter-gatherer peoples, indicates that our ancestors' lives may not have been so 'nasty, brutish and short' as we might have thought. Our ancestors would have suffered from infectious diseases, as do contemporary hunter-gatherer peoples, either in epidemics (where unusual infections occur and subsequently become widespread but are limited spatially and temporally) or from sporadic episodes of infectious diseases (where a few instances might occur now and then). Our pre-historic ancestors would also have been exposed to similar zoonotic infections as are non-human primates (Armelagos et al., 2005), yet their healthy and well-balanced diet may well have strengthened their ability to counter them. However, low group size meant that 'crowd' diseases such as measles and smallpox could not be supported, nor was there much trade between groups to allow the opportunity to introduce new infections, and without permanent buildings, there was little opportunity for refuse to accumulate and harbour infectious disease vectors such as rats (Roberts & Cox, 2003).

The switch from hunter-gathering to agricultural settlements would have led to increasing food supplies and a resulting rise in human populations. Ironically, the switch to agriculture and settlement led to a smaller-bodied, less well-nourished and more disease-prone people, who would have been vulnerable to harvest failure. Living in settlements would also have increased proximity to animals and their pathogens, as well as proximity to human and animal faeces and vermin. Endemic diseases, such as tuberculosis, leprosy, smallpox, measles, mumps, whooping cough, scarlet fever and diphtheria, became possible only with a stable and large enough population to support them. Trade would have subsequently facilitated their spread. The first geographical areas where population density reached from ten to 100 times that of the hunter-gatherers were in Jericho and the Fertile crescent, which were also the places where the first Biblical 'plagues' occurred (Crawford, 2007).

The Roman period saw rural to urban migration occurring across Europe, providing the opportunity for people to contract new diseases. Archaeological skeletal evidence from Britain in this period indicates evidence of wasting poliomyelitis, leprosy and tuberculosis. Although the Romans have a reputation for hygiene, this was probably little more than skin deep, and archaeological evidence indicates that bed bugs, lice, intestinal worms and black rats were widespread in Roman towns. After the fall of the Roman Empire around 410AD, there was ongoing clearance of land across Europe, allowing areas to become marshy and wet, leading to an increased incidence of malaria. Towns and trade continued to develop in the medieval period, with densely packed buildings and filthy, poor and contaminated living environments; vermin, lice and fly infestations; and polluted water supplies. In 664 in England there was an occurrence of a 'plague' of some kind that lasted for fifty years, with further outbreaks of 'pestilence' occurring between the eighth and eleventh centuries (Roberts & Cox, 2003).

In later medieval Europe, as food production rose, so the population continued to grow, but by the early fourteenth century the population had outstripped the available food supply. The famine that resulted would have exacerbated the impact of the Black Death of 1348–9, which killed as many as half the population in many countries in Europe. Medieval Europeans lived in crowded housing and close to their animals, leading to exposure to zoonotic infections such as tuberculosis and brucellosis (which was called undulating fever, reflecting its recurrent nature). Drinking water would have been contaminated from wells dug near to cesspits, and from sewerage dumped in the streets. Most people would have possessed only a few items of clothing, which would have led to the persistence of parasites such as fleas, ticks and lice. Ironically, whilst such poor hygiene was a potential source of infection, it would also have led to higher resistance to common bacterial infections (Roberts & Cox, 2003).

Between 1485 and 1551, a new epidemic of 'sweating sickness' appeared in Europe, the exact nature of which remains unknown, although it has been unconvincingly identified as typhus, influenza, malaria and meningitis. As it particularly affected the upper classes, it has been suggested that it was a type of haemorrhagic fever dependent on a tick vector, possibly from deer hunting and consumption of infected meat (Roberts & Cox, 2003). Between 1493 and 1530, a virulent syphilis epidemic spread through Europe. The syphilis epidemic followed soon after the discovery of the New World by Columbus, and so led to the (contested) notion that it was introduced from there. In the Americas, only turkeys, duck, guinea pigs, llamas and alpaca were farmed, none of which were likely to donate microbes to humans (Crawford, 2007). So with the exception of tuberculosis, which archaeological evidence from Native American ossuaries shows was present in pre-Columbian America (Ryan, 1992), the Native Americans had no resistance to Old World crowd diseases. Around the same time in the New World, Old World diseases such as smallpox, measles, mumps and chickenpox were decimating the indigenous populations.

In Europe in the sixteenth and seventeenth centuries, there were numerous epidemics of typhus fever, typhoid fever and smallpox. Smallpox seems rarely to have been lethal in Britain before 1630, but after the last great plague of 1665, a new or more virulent strain of smallpox seems to have evolved or been introduced. Smallpox reached its peak following the rapid urbanisation of the early industrial revolution of the eighteenth century (Crawford, 2007). National statistics of several European countries indicate that smallpox was directly responsible for between 8 and 20 per cent of all deaths in the eighteenth century (Bonanni, 1999).

Variation – the inoculation into the skin of healthy people of material from pustules of those suffering with smallpox to induce immunity – was reported in China and in India as early as the tenth century, and Egypt in the thirteenth century. But it is Lady Mary Wortley-Montagu who is widely credited with introducing variolation to Britain from Turkey in 1721. She had been left severely scarred following smallpox and, convinced of the efficacy of variolation, successfully had her own children variolated. Her success was subsequently advertised and the practice became widespread (Fenner et al., 1988). Naturally acquired smallpox carried a one in six risk of death, however, variolation itself carried a one in 50 risk that the person would develop smallpox and die. By 1765, refinements in the technique of injecting the virus had reduced mortality to less than one in 500 (Boylston, 2002).

Edward Jenner, an English country doctor, had noticed that milkmaids were rarely pockmarked. There was a vague notion amongst country people that the reason milkmaids did not contract smallpox was that they were protected by the similar, milder disease of cattle, cowpox, which they came into contact with when milking. Jenner experimented with the inoculation of cowpox pustules into healthy people to protect them against smallpox, and then inoculation with the smallpox virus itself into those he had already inoculated with cowpox to see if cowpox provided immunity. He called his procedure 'vaccination', from the Latin for cow, *vacca*, to distinguish it from variolation.

In 1798, when smallpox was at its most destructive stage in Europe, he published *An inquiry into the causes and effects of the variolae vaccinae, a disease discovered in some of the western counties of England, particularly Gloucestershire and known by the name of cowpox*. Jenner's discovery was quickly adopted throughout Europe and spread around the world, and there is substantial evidence that the decline in mortality in Europe in the first decade of the nineteenth century was in large part attributable to it (Bonanni, 1999).

In 1840, The British Parliament passed an Act that forbade the practice of variolation, and in 1841 a supplementary Act was introduced which enabled cowpox-type vaccine to be made available to those who could not afford it. Despite its success, from the beginning of the eighteenth century there were religious objections to the practice of both variolation and later to vaccination. It was argued that variolation and vaccination thwarted of the will of God, and people should accept what God had set out for them – to resist was to turn away from God, and by doing so ensure damnation (Spier, 2002).

The successes of public health campaigns

By about 1800, leprosy and plague had all but disappeared from Europe, and malaria and smallpox were declining. 'Ague' was a major killer cited on Bills of Mortality in the second half of the seventeenth century. As with many historical diseases, it is unclear what modern disease ague corresponds to, although it has been ascribed to malaria. Epidemics of communicable disease in Europe were less serious and less widespread in the eighteenth than in the seventeenth century, although influenza and a by now less virulent form of syphilis were still common. There was also an increase in the prevalence of childhood killers such as scarlet fever, whooping cough (pertussis), measles and diphtheria (Roberts & Cox, 2003).

In most northern European countries there was a fall in death rates from the end of the eighteenth century due to a decrease in deaths of children over one year old. The death rates of infants below one year was dependent on the extent to which they were breast fed, and their survival rate improved before the modern economic growth period of the second part of the nineteenth century. Research carried out in Sweden in this period has found that children over one year old, particularly from poor families, were more vulnerable (than breast-fed infants) to economic fluctuations and were more likely to die in years following an extremely poor harvest, though whether they died from lack of resistance to common diseases due to malnutrition, or because of the spread of less common diseases during migration to seek work is unclear (Bengtsson, 1999).

The trend of rural to urban migration continued in the eighteenth century, particularly in Britain in the early years of the industrial revolution. Mortality remained high due to the risk of famine, as well as death from infectious diseases, particularly due to poor hygiene, contaminated drinking water and inadequate sewerage. The rise in population, overcrowding in urban slums and exploitation of labour that characterised the industrial revolution facilitated the great epidemic scourges of the nineteenth century: TB and cholera.

TB was, and to a certain extent still is, associated with the artistic people who suffered from it: the Brontës, Shelley, Keats, Lawrence, Balzac, Chekhov, Kafka, Chopin and so on. Before the contagiousness of TB was established in 1882, most people believed that 'consumption' was hereditary and could only be improved or cured by a change of climate. The French resort of Nice, for example,

> ... was the most fashionable rendezvous [in the nineteenth century] for those who tried to dodge death every winter by escaping from northern frosts. At the Opera House, performances of the 'cooing, phthisical' [phthisis meaning TB] music of the Romantic Era nightly attracted throngs of corpse-like consumptives. The young women were smartly dressed and lavishly jewelled, but so pale beneath their curls that their faces appeared to be powdered with 'scrapings of bones'. Indeed, it seemed to one witness as if cemeteries were not closed at night and allowed the dead to escape. (Dubos & Dubos, 1952: 20)

As so many famous artistic people suffered with TB, it was thought that the disease afflicted those who were more sensitive or artistic. Its prevalence also influenced the fashions of the day; for pale, emaciated ethereal women, and for the high neckerchiefs worn by men to hide the visible scrofula (swollen and discharging tuberculous lymph glands in the neck). Even a consumptive cough was considered fascinating by the early Victorians (Dubos & Dubos, 1952). Although upper and middle-class consumptives were thought to be beautiful and artistic, this concept did not extend to the urban poor affected by the disease, who were regarded as miserable and frightening. 'In the course of the nineteenth century, tuberculosis thus became bound up in two successive chains of signifiers: passion, the idleness and the luxury of the sanatorium, and pleasure-filled life 'apart' on the one hand ... the dank and airless slum, and exhaustion leading to an atrocious agony on the other' (Herzlich & Pierret, 1984: 28).

The industrialised countries of the nineteenth century also saw repeated and terrifying epidemics of two intestinal diseases: cholera and typhoid. Although cholera had circulated continuously on the Indian subcontinent for many centuries, it was unknown in Europe or America before the 1800s. Until the British entered India in the mid 1700s, cholera would have been relatively mild, intermittent and local phenomenon. Only after the East India Company took control of Bengal in 1757 did cholera cause epidemics and it spread outward from India after 1817 as a result of trade (Alcabes, 2009). Although statistically it killed less people than TB, the social significance of 'Asiatic' cholera was tremendous. In 1830, a cholera epidemic originating in India swept across Russia. The following year it moved across Europe, reaching America in 1832. Victims produced huge amounts of 'rice-water' diarrhoea, and sufferers usually died within a few days.

In many ways Asiatic cholera was directly responsible for the birth of the public health movement in Britain. Works such as Edwin Chadwick's 1842 *Report on the Sanitary Condition of the Labouring Population of Great Britain* and Friedrich Engels's 1845 *Condition of the Working Class in England* provided detailed accounts of how living conditions in the urban slums contributed to the spread of infectious diseases. Known colloquially as 'fever nests', the Victorian slums lacked ventilation, fresh water and adequate sanitation, were severely overcrowded, encouraging epidemics and exacerbating disorders arising from malnutrition such as rickets and scurvy (O'Conner, 2000).

Chadwick's report in particular argued that miasmas generated by organic filth were responsible for generating disease. The 'sanitarians' thus argued that the streets should be cleansed and flushed and water carriage and sewerage systems introduced. The sanitarians' success in reducing the incidence of cholera confirmed for them their belief in the miasmic theory of disease (see Chapter 6). It was not until John Snow's work in the 1850s that cholera was linked to contaminated water supplies. Cholera for Europeans thus became an issue for consolidating the successes of liberal capitalism, and became a focus for addressing the problems of poverty and the poor. In the USA, thinking about cholera was viewed through a more religious lens, being associated not only with poor crowded neighbourhoods (and therefore with the Irish), but also with impiety, impurity and intemperance (Alcabes, 2009).

Despite the earlier successful adoption of Jenner's discovery of vaccination, the really significant decrease in mortality from smallpox followed the compulsory vaccination of infants before they reached the age of four. This was introduced in Britain by an 1853 Act of Parliament, with a fine of 20 shillings for those parents who refused (Spier, 2002). The act led to violent riots in several English towns. The anti-vaccine movement was started in 1854 with a pamphlet, written by John Gibbs, entitled 'Our Medical Liberties'. An even stronger act in 1867 sanctioned non-vaccination of infants with imprisonment for 14 days. This bolstered the anti-vaccination movement and a weekly magazine *The Anti-Vaccinator* appeared from 1869. By this time the movement was concerned with the autonomy of the individual. Anti-vaccinationists argued that the law was being brought into disrepute by criminalising people who had not committed a crime. Vaccinators were held to be trampling the rights of parents to their children, who were considered their property (Spier, 2002).

Similar anti-vaccination movements flourished elsewhere. In Stockholm, for example, anti-vaccination sentiment had led vaccination rates to fall to just over 40 per cent by 1872, while they approached 90 per cent in the rest of Sweden. A major epidemic in the city in 1874 led to widespread vaccination and an end to further epidemics. In the USA, widespread smallpox vaccination in the early part of the nineteenth century had contained the disease and vaccination fell into disuse. The consequent susceptibility of the unvaccinated population led to its reappearance in the USA in the 1870s. As individual states tried to enact legislation or enforce existing vaccination laws, American anti-vaccination leagues were set up. In Britain, an anti-vaccination demonstration by 100,000 people in Leicester in 1885 led to the establishment of a Royal Commission, and a new Vaccination Act followed in 1898, which included a conscience clause to allow for a right to refuse vaccination (Wolfe & Sharp, 2002).

There is some evidence that smallpox in England was anyway becoming slowly less virulent throughout the first half of the nineteenth century, with a steadily falling death rate. Vaccination was the principal feature of smallpox preventative policy in Britain up to the later 1860s; however, compulsory vaccination was inadequate in itself as it did not incur lifelong immunity. Between 1870 and 1872 Britain saw the worst smallpox epidemic of the century, with 44,500 smallpox deaths, including nearly 8,000 in London alone. This led to the establishment of a 'stamping out' policy, with isolation in hospital of all cases of smallpox and tracing and vaccination of contacts. As a result, smallpox was virtually absent from London by the 1890s. There was an outbreak in 1901, but by August 1902 it had been virtually eliminated (Hardy, 1993). An increasing acceptance of the governments' role in public health in

Western countries led to the slow collapse of the anti-vaccination movement, although as discussed in Chapter 6, it was to re-emerge in the late
twentieth century.

The huge growth in population in developed countries from the eighteenth century onwards was essentially due to a reduction in deaths
from infectious diseases, rather than from an increase in birth rates,
which had been falling in most developed countries since records began.
The decline in both morbidity (illness) and mortality from infectious
diseases is usually credited to the progress in medical knowledge, particularly following the discoveries of Louis Pasteur and Robert Koch after
the 1880s, but as McKeown (1976) in his seminal book *The Modern Rise
of Population* demonstrated, the explanation for the growth in the population of developed countries lay in improvements in nutrition and the
environment, rather than in 'medical progress'. Improvements in nutrition due to greater food supplies and the consequent rise in standards
of health and immunity to infection led to the population in England
and Wales trebling between 1700 and 1850. From the second half of the
nineteenth century, there were also improvements in the environment,
so that intestinal infections had been substantially reduced due to the
introduction of water purification and sewerage disposal and improved
food hygiene, particularly with regard to milk. Between 1838 and 1935,
specific *medical* measures made only a small contribution to the total
decline in the death rates from smallpox, syphilis, tetanus, diphtheria,
diarrhoeal diseases and some surgical conditions.

The golden age of medicine

The period between the 1870s and the 1970s has been dubbed 'the
golden age of medicine'. Before the discoveries of Pasteur and Koch
gained widespread acceptance around the late 1870s, many of the most
brilliant medical practitioners of the time still opposed the germ theory
of disease. Most doctors had thought of health as a harmony between
the individual and the environment, and between various forces at work
in the body. Before the discovery of specific microbes for different diseases, doctors thought that one disease could develop into another, and
did not accept the idea that each disease was separate and had a specific
cause (Dubos, 1959).

The twentieth century saw many heroic medical breakthroughs and
successes in medicine and drug therapies for non-infective causes, in

anaesthetics and surgery. However, arguably the breakthroughs that affected the most people, and had the most impact in terms of creating the mood of optimism around 'medical progress', were those surrounding infectious diseases. Koch developed practical techniques of bacteriology in 1877, and applied his techniques to tuberculosis. Between 1875 and the early 1890s, Pasteur and his followers identified around 50 specific agents of infectious diseases affecting humans and animals, including anthrax, typhoid fever, cholera, plague, malaria, diphtheria, tetanus, *Escherichia coli,* influenza and dysentery.

The development of antimicrobial drugs and vaccinations that followed in the early twentieth century built on these foundations. One of the first benefits from the discoveries of bacteriology was their practical application by Joseph Lister, then a surgeon in Glasgow, who sought to apply Pasteur's discoveries of germ theory to his own field. Through his experiments with carbolic acid solution swabbed on wounds, published in *The Lancet* in 1867, Lister found that he could markedly reduced the incidence of gangrene (Winslow, 1943).

In 1910, Paul Ehrlich discovered the first drug to be successful against syphilis – Salvarsan – with Prontosil following in 1935. These first antimicrobial drugs, the sulphonamides, were used also to treat pneumonia, meningitis, gastrointestinal and urinary infections, and streptococcal infections such as puerperal fever, which was still responsible for the deaths of two in every 1,000 women in labour up to the 1930s (Kingston, 2000). Ehrlich coined the term 'magic bullets' to describe the potential of new drugs that promised, as he put it, 'to strike only the objects against which they are targeted'. This metaphor, together with that of the 'wonder drug', became widely used in the 1930s and 1940s to capture the optimism and promise of the new 'golden age of medicine' (Bud, 2006).

In the period between 1900 and 1918, there was a steep decline in mortality from infectious diseases throughout the developed world. Never before in the history of the world had people enjoyed such good health. Trust in medicine had become so elevated as almost to reach the level of a new religion (Tognotti, 2003).

However, bacteriologists were impotent in the face of the 'Spanish' influenza pandemic (worldwide epidemic) of 1918–19. It is estimated that the virus caused acute illness in over a quarter of the world's population (500 million people) and the death toll from the pandemic has been estimated at 40 million people. However, these figures are likely to be a significant underestimate, as more recent studies suggest that the estimated global mortality of the pandemic may be something in the order of 50 million people. Even this vast figure may still be substantially lower than the real death toll, which may have been as high as 100 million (Johnson & Mueller, 2002).

The very wide geographical spread of deaths in the 1918 influenza pandemic in such a short period, and the absence of air travel at the time, suggest that the disease had migrated around the globe prior to this time. Evidence points to the epidemic having been 'seeded' in two British army camps in Etaples, France and Aldershot, England in 1916. Restrictions on travel during the war would have also protracted the epidemic, and then the demobilisation of late 1918 would have provided the circumstances for the virus to be carried around the world by demobilised troops, with arrival parties at home possibly exacerbating the situation by providing opportunities for the virus to spread. Rather than a westward spread from the east, there is evidence that the virus spread eastward from Europe towards China (Oxford, 2001). Wartime censorship in the French, British and German newspapers meant that nothing was printed that might damage morale. Spain actually had very few cases, but unlike other governments, the Spanish government did not censor the press. Therefore it was only Spanish newspapers that were publishing accounts of the spread of the disease, and the pandemic became known as 'Spanish' influenza (Barry, 2005).

The exceptionally high mortality rate in the 1918–19 influenza pandemic was mostly caused by bacterial pneumonia secondary to the viral infection, frequently causing death within a few days of infection. The really unique feature of the 1918 pandemic, and one which remains unexplained, was the high death rate among young adults aged 20–40, who usually have a very low death rate from influenza, while, inexplicably, those in the 5–14 age group accounted for a large proportion of cases, but had a comparably very low mortality rate (Taubenberger et al., 2001).

In Summer 1928, at St Mary's Hospital in Paddington, London, Alexander Fleming famously prepared a number of Petri dish cultures of staphylococci before leaving them while he went on holiday. When he returned he found a growth of mould around which colonies of microbes had not developed. Fleming thus discovered the antibiotic properties of penicillin. However, he could only produce the penicillin in very small quantities and thus took it no further as a treatment for infections. Nevertheless, he did find a valuable laboratory use for it in inhibiting the growth of other bacteria on cultured influenza swabs, thereby aiding the diagnosis of influenza.

After the disastrous impact of the 1918 pandemic on the military, the development of influenza vaccine was given priority. In 1933 the virus that caused influenza was discovered. In the run up to the Second World War, Macfarlane Burnet, working with the Australian army, concentrated on the development of a vaccine using live influenza virus, while the US military favoured an attenuated vaccine (using inactivated or killed virus). By 1943, results in the USA were sufficiently encouraging to dissuade further live vaccine development and methods for large-scale production of attenuated vaccine were developed. The WHO set up a global influenza surveillance network in 1948 (Kitler et al., 2002). Fleming's virtually unique strain of penicillin was kept in production in tiny amounts, which later became crucial for the development by Florey and Chain of the first large scale antibiotics (Kingston, 2000).

As well as the development of a vaccine for influenza, there were other major successes against infectious diseases due to the development of vaccines prior to the introduction of antibiotics in the late 1940s. The first modern vaccine was for typhoid and was tested on a large scale on British and French soldiers in the First World War. This was followed by vaccines for tetanus in 1921, diphtheria in 1923 and yellow fever in 1932 (Moulin, 2000). After the 1920s, the viral causes of measles, mumps, poliomyelitis, dengue fever and the common cold were discovered (Winslow, 1943).

Typhoid fever (which, like cholera, is bacterial and spread by the faecal–oral route) and typhus fever have similar symptoms, and it was only in 1909 that it was discovered that typhus fever was a separate disease transmitted by body lice. Later again it was discovered that typhus is one of a family of Rickettsia diseases and that it is transmitted not only by lice, but also by rat fleas. Since the 1870s, typhus had been declining in Europe, and in the decade before the First World War, the only Western country with any considerable typhus incidence was Ireland. However, because of the conditions of war, there was an outbreak in 1914–15 in Europe, which killed 150,000 people in six months. In the social upheaval following the creation of the Soviet Union between 1917 and 1921, there were an estimated 25 million cases and 2.5–3 million deaths in the territories controlled by the Soviet Republic (Zinsser, 1935). A vaccine against typhus was developed by Hans Zinsser in 1932. Vaccination, together with antibiotics and the control of rats and lice, combined to reduce the incidence of typhus throughout the world, although further outbreaks during the

Second World War killed many, particularly in the Nazi concentration camps.

As well as the discovery of the insect vector of typhus fever, the early years of the twentieth century also saw the discovery and acceptance that mosquitoes were the carriers of both yellow fever and malaria. Yellow fever was imported into the New World from Africa in slave ships and appeared in the USA 35 times between 1702 and 1800; between 1800 and 1879 there were epidemics in all but two years. The scourge of centuries was wiped out promptly by controlling the mosquito carrier. This enabled the completion of the Panama Canal in 1914, the construction of which had been repeatedly sabotaged by outbreaks of yellow fever and malaria amongst the construction workers. By 1929, the last known centres of yellow fever in the Americas were under control, although animal reservoirs in wild animals meant that eradicating yellow fever entirely was untenable (Winslow, 1943).

In the 1930s, the eradication of malaria-carrying mosquitoes in Brazil began to be carried out, and by 1941 all *Anopheles gambiae* mosquitoes had been eradicated from that country. The following year Bolivia also announced the eradication of *Aedes aegypti* mosquitoes. These successes led the WHO to support similar programmes in many countries, and led to the goal of eradication in many other infectious disease projects (Cockburn, 1963).

In 1936, Ernst Chain found Fleming's 1929 paper on penicillin and persuaded his fellow researcher at Oxford, Howard Florey, that they should try to address the problem that had defeated Fleming. After encouraging animal experiments, they managed to manufacture enough penicillin to do some human trials on surgical patients who had been given up for lost by their doctors. The 'unbelievable' results from these trials were reported in the medical journal *The Lancet* in August 1940 (Kingston, 2000).

However, the problem remained of how to manufacture enough penicillin to carry out full-scale human trials. Eventually Chain and Florey decided that the British effort would never succeed in producing sufficient quantities of penicillin. Florey visited the USA, and within a few weeks of his arrival the USA had increased the production capacity for the drug by a factor of 12. In March 1942, there was enough penicillin to treat only one human case, but by August 1943, 500 had been treated. By 1944, enough was produced to treat all the needy casualties of the Normandy invasion, by which time limited distribution had begun to US civilians (Kingston, 2000). After the end of the war, penicillin gradually became widely available to civilians in the USA and Britain (Bud, 1998).

As well as tackling infections following trauma and surgery, the other great success of antibiotics was against 'venereal disease', as penicillin could cure syphilis completely with just one dose. As a result of penicillin, by the mid-1950s it seemed that venereal infections could no longer be considered a major public health threat. However, by the late 1950s the incidence of venereal disease had begun to climb once again. In the USA between 1965 and 1975 cases of gonorrhoea more than tripled, rising to over one million per year. In 1980 alone, more than two million cases of gonorrhoea were reported in the USA, and a small but growing number of these were resistant to standard antibiotic therapy (Brandt, 1985).

Penicillin however, had no effect on TB. TB had in fact began to regress spontaneously in Europe during the course of the nineteenth and early twentieth centuries, because of improved living conditions and general health, although contemporaries were unaware of this (Herzlich & Pierret, 1984). Decline in the prevalence of TB in Europe was also due to vaccination, following the 1919 development by Calmette and Guerin of a weakened form of TB bacteria that had been tested in animals, the bacilli Calmette-Guerin (BCG). The USA rejected the BCG vaccine, a reflection of its antipathy towards universal health interventions which might strengthen the role of the state, and subvert the self-improvement ethos of the New Deal, and at the same time draw attention to the persistence of TB (Gandy, 2003).

In 1930, 90,000 people in the USA still died of TB, as did 66,000 in France, and 50,000 in England and Wales (Ryan, 1992). Although there was a downward trend in mortality, the two world wars had a severe, if geographically uneven, upward impact on TB mortality trends in Europe (Smallman-Raynor & Cliff, 2003). The first effective anti-TB treatment, streptomycin, was introduced for clinical use in 1946 and was soon followed by other drugs: para-aminosalicylic acid (PAS) in 1950, isoniazid and pyrazinamide in 1952, ethambutol in 1963 and rifampin in 1966 (Reichman & Tanne, 2002). Although resistance to these drugs was soon reported when given individually, trials showed that when given together, the drugs could completely cure TB. By 1960, the WHO and the United Nations were able to propose the complete eradication of TB from the world.

In Europe and North America in particular, 'the golden age of medicine' also saw huge advances in controlling common childhood diseases. Scarlet fever and measles had been decreasing in virulence throughout Western Europe and North America both in terms of incidence and mortality since the late nineteenth century. However, once infected with measles, there is still no treatment, and before the 1960s quarantine was the only protection against it.

The attenuated measles virus vaccine was developed by John Franklin Enders from Harvard and was successfully tested in the USA in 1961. It had become widely available in the USA by 1963. Before the introduction of the vaccine there were four million cases of measles in the USA per year, with 48,000 requiring hospitalisation and 5,000 deaths. 4,000 of the more serious cases led to encephalitis, and 1,000 of those were left with permanent brain damage and deafness. By the time the measles vaccine was introduced into the UK in 1968, there were less than 100 cases a year, with two deaths. By the 1980s measles was rare in developed countries and the WHO stepped up global efforts against the disease (Oldstone, 1998).

The other great medical success story in relation to childhood infections was the 'conquest of polio'. Ironically, the epidemics of polio in developed countries in the twentieth century were a result of improved standards of personal hygiene and purer food and water, which resulted in a substantial reduction in other diseases, but caused a dramatic increase in polio, as there was a reduction in the chances of exposure to natural infection. Although there were epidemics of polio around the world, between 1919 and 1934 over half the reported cases were in North America. Cases increased steadily in the USA until in 1952 they reached an unprecedented 57,628. In 1955, the discovery of the 'safe effective and potent' attenuated Salk polio vaccine was announced. Church bells were rung in some American towns at the good news and Salk became an overnight celebrity (Gould, 1995).

In Britain there was never the same urgency about polio, as it was a comparatively rare disease until after the Second World War. Britain had its first large epidemic in 1947, when 7,776 cases were reported. Immunisation was introduced for children in Britain in 1956, and a campaign was launched to encourage the wider take-up of the Salk vaccine in 1958. The action of the attenuated Salk vaccine prevented polio causing damage, but did not prevent the spread of the infection. Sabin's live oral vaccine, by contrast, worked in a similar way to the 'wild virus' itself, spreading polio in a harmless form. Britain endorsed the Sabin vaccine in 1962, after it had been used in Russia in 1959–60 to successfully immunise 100 million people (Gould, 1995).

Such successes led to the possibility being raised of eradication of several other diseases throughout the world. Between the two world wars, The Rockefeller Foundation established ambitious plans for the eradication of diseases such as syphilis and TB (Moulin, 2000). However, it was the eradication of smallpox that gave a concrete form to these utopian dreams.

By the early 1950s, endemic smallpox had been eliminated from North America and Europe. At the 12th World Health Assembly in 1959, the USSR successfully proposed a resolution calling for worldwide eradication of smallpox. By 1967, Brazil was the only South American country where smallpox was endemic. There were substantial gains in smallpox control in Asia between 1959 and 1966, particularly the elimination of smallpox from China in 1961, although the disease remained rampant in India and in 27 of the 47 countries of Africa. In 1967, the Intensified Smallpox Eradication Programme was instituted by the WHO, leading to a rapid fall in the number of developing countries with endemic smallpox. The eradication of smallpox from the Indian subcontinent was achieved by 1975. By 1976, the only remaining endemic country was Ethiopia, where smallpox persisted and from where it spread to Somalia. Smallpox was eventually eradicated from the Horn of Africa at the end of 1977 (Fenner et al., 1988).

The successful eradication of smallpox led to the political will to tackle other infectious diseases on a global level. In 1974, the WHO, together with the United Nations Children's Fund (UNICEF), established the Expanded Programme on Immunization (EPI). The aim was to provide all children in their first year with basic immunisation, including vaccines against diphtheria, tetanus, poliomyelitis, whooping cough, and later measles, under the banner 'Health for All in the Year 2000' (World Health Organization, 1978). As a result of EPI the yearly incidence of measles fell from its 1960s level of about 135 million cases, with over six million deaths, to 1.9 million deaths by 1987, and only 875,000 deaths by 1990 (Kaufmann, 2009). By the 1990s basic vaccine coverage had risen from 5 per cent to 80 per cent of the annual birth cohort, saving three million lives annually.

This success in turn led to speculation that other diseases might also be eradicated from the world. The NIH hosted a conference in May 1980 that considered the eradication of several diseases. The three that received most attention were measles, poliomyelitis and yaws (a chronic and highly infectious tropical skin disease) (Stetten, 1980). The effort to eradicate poliomyelitis was launched in 1988 by the World Health Assembly, and included National Immunization Days (NID) in polio-endemic countries, supported by international agencies, countries and supported by international agencies and the private sector, particularly Rotary International (Widdus, 1999).

The 'diseases of civilisation'

With the eradication of smallpox, the triumph of medicine against infectious diseases seemed, if not complete, then at least in sight. The 1970s saw a number of critical voices being raised against medicine: for example Michel Foucault's critique of the power relations in medical discourse (Foucault, 1973); Ivan Illich's critique of the medicalisation of pain and death (Illich, 1976); and the feminist critique of the medicalisation of childbirth. Yet few could argue against the triumphalism of biomedicine in the sphere of infectious diseases. As discussed above, the epidemiological transition model, itself a product of the 1970s, argued that a new transition was occurring, where due to the continuing decline from infectious diseases, mortality would continue to decline, and as we lived longer, we would increasingly succumb to the so-called 'diseases of civilisation' such as heart disease and cancer.

Evidence for this shift in public perceptions can be found in Herzlich & Pierret's (1984) *Illness and Self in Society*, which describes social scientific studies carried out in France in the period 1960 to 1980. In it, they argue that '[i]n France at least, 1960 represents a turning point, a pivot between a past dominated by infectious disease – poliomyelitis was its last embodiment, and tuberculosis is its symbol to this day – and a present in which illness has definitely assumed a different face' (Herzlich & Pierret, 1984 : 46). This different face of illness was cancer – the only 'real' disease worth talking about; 'the face of death': 'THE illness of our time'.

Up to the end of the nineteenth century, evidence shows that people were more afraid of infectious diseases than they were of cancer. For example, a fascinating survey published in *The American Journal of Psychology* in 1896 (Scott, 1896) asked respondents (n = 226) about their notions on the subject of old age, death and future life. The researchers asked the adult respondents about what they feared most when they were children, and found that the order of what they most feared was:

smallpox; lockjaw (tetanus); consumption (TB); hydrophobia (rabies); railroad accidents; diphtheria; drowning; fire; leprosy; earthquakes; lightning; pneumonia; miscellaneous accidents; and only then cancer, which ranked equally with yellow fever and cyclones. Only tornadoes, the end of the world, and fear of being the last person alive were ranked lower than cancer (Scott, 1896).

However, concern about cancer grew through the early years of the twentieth century, when increasing rates of cancer were blamed on it being a 'disease of civilisation'. *Civilisation* here originally has a cluster of meanings around urbanisation, insufficient or excess diet, affluence, climate, the reversal of sex roles, changing morals, promiscuity, psychological causes and so on. Later in the twentieth century, the notion of cancer as a 'disease of *civilisation'* in the sense of 'good living' or 'excess' was succeeded by the narrower notion of civilisation meaning *environment.* Pipe smoking was recognised as a cause of cancer of the lip in the eighteenth century, and by 1915 the relation to cancer of the mouth was in little doubt. The link to lung cancer was postulated in the 1920s, and becoming increasingly clear that the chances of getting cancer were related to environmental causes. By 1950, Doll and Hill showed that people who smoked more than 25 cigarettes a day were about 50 times more likely than non-smokers to die of lung cancer (Proctor, 1995).

By the 1930s, the dominant view was that overall cancer rates were increasing. This prompted, in 1937, a change in the context of US cancer research with the passing of a National Cancer Institute Act and, with it, the creation of a new federal agency, The Cancer Institute. After the Second World War, vastly increased funds were made available to cancer researchers and cancer research was scaled up, meriting the title 'Big Science'. Founded in 1945, the Sloan-Kettering Institute in Manhattan quickly became the largest ever private cancer research institute in the USA, with a budget in 1950 of US$1.8 million, twice the expenditure on cancer research in the entire country in 1937. From the mid-1950s, research into chemotherapy for cancer expanded rapidly. There was a feeling that the USA should launch a directed, nationally integrated attempt to find a cure for cancer, along the lines of the wartime projects such as the development of penicillin (Bud, 1978).

The 1960s and 1970s also saw increasing concern about environmental damage and pollution, particularly after the publication of Rachel Carson's *Silent Spring* (Carson, 1962), which popularised the notion of environmental damage causing cancer. In 1971, President Nixon launched his 'War on Cancer'. In his second State of the Union address, Nixon said:

> I will also ask for an appropriation of an extra US$100 million to launch an intensive campaign to find a cure for cancer, and I will ask later for whatever additional funds can effectively be used. The time has come in America when the same kind of concentrated effort that split the atom and took man to the moon should be turned toward conquering this dread disease. Let us make a total national commitment to achieve this goal.

Some reservations were voiced about Nixon's 'War on Cancer', particularly from those who felt that the biggest killer in the USA, heart disease, would have been a more appropriate target for research funding (Chubin & Studer, 1978). However, Nixon's optimism was based on the acknowledgement that the war on infectious diseases was nearly won, and reflected the era's faith in science and technology. If President Kennedy could send a man to the moon, then Nixon's era would be marked by a cure for cancer (Proctor, 1995).

In fact, the incidence in most types of cancer had not increased in the USA during the twentieth century, with the exception of those related to smoking. At the same time there had been a big drop in gastrointestinal cancers, perhaps related to a move away from consumption of smoked and salted meats and fish (Urquhart & Heilmann, 1984). Cancer, and even more so cardiovascular disease, had risen up the table of causes in death in developed countries simply because deaths from infectious diseases had fallen (see tables below).

Nevertheless, from the 1950s to the 1980s, cancer was the most feared and stigmatised disease. The very word cancer was awesome, unspeakable. The metaphoric force of cancer: the dread, the shame, the guilt that accompanied it, filled the same symbolic space that for a previous generation had been occupied by syphilis and TB. When Susan Sontag wrote her essay *Illness as Metaphor* (Sontag, 1978), she was facing an apparently terminal cancer prognosis herself. While it still retains its brilliance, with hindsight Sontag's essay can be seen as a marker of the last moment when cancer would be feared above all other illnesses.

A number of new infectious diseases appeared in the 1970s, which many writers have retrospectively dubbed 'the gathering storm' – see, for example, Laurie Garrett's (1995) *The Coming Plague*. Yet given the focus on cancer at the time, these new infectious diseases were thought relatively unimportant, or at least manageable. The 1976 Ebola epidemic in Africa for example, was largely ignored by the Western press at the time (see Chapter 5).

Also in 1976, an outbreak of a severe form of pneumonia during the annual American Legion convention in Philadelphia led to 221 cases and 34 deaths. The epidemic was found to be caused by a newly discovered *Legionella pneumonophilia*, (although investigators retrospectively identified the pathogen from stored samples from earlier outbreaks from as far back as 1957). Legionnaires' disease struck those with compromised immune systems and underlying medical conditions, such as the elderly, or people with chronic heart or lung conditions. The organism has since been isolated from natural freshwater environments but has rarely been implicated as a source of human disease except in human-made environments (Fry & Besser, 2002).

In the same year a 'swine flu' epidemic was threatened, when a US soldier stationed at Fort Dix, New Jersey, died mysteriously from a strain of influenza virus. Testing revealed that another six troops were infected with the virus, which was similar to one causing disease in swine. Concerned there had been a major antigenic shift in the influenza virus, the US government introduced a US$135 million plan to inoculate every American. When the news of Legionnaires' disease broke later that year, the news shocked the US Congress into approval of the *National Swine Flu Immunization Program 1976*, which waived liability in the case of adverse events following vaccination. The vaccination programme started in October, and President Ford and his family were vaccinated live on television. Almost immediately there were reports of deaths and adverse reactions to the vaccine, and the vaccination programme was abruptly stopped in December 1976. In the event, only 13 mild cases of influenza developed at Fort Dix and the strain was not found elsewhere (Levy & Fischetti, 2003).

At the end of the 1970s, two other infections generated media storms: In 1980 the CDC was informed of a sudden surge in acute bacterial infections related to tampon use, which became known as 'toxic shock syndrome'. The other big story of the time was the moral panic surrounding the rise in genital herpes, which by 1980 affected approximately 25 million Americans, 16.4 per cent of all Americans between the ages of 15 and 74 (Johnson et al., 1989). However, rather than denting the optimism that biomedicine could conquer infectious diseases, the scares around Legionnaires' disease, toxic shock syndrome and genital herpes seemed to confirm that biomedical science could successfully tackle whatever new threats arose.

It is difficult to get a precise statistical picture of mortality and morbidity from infectious disease as infections may be secondary to other events, such as peritonitis, and infections are also important contributors to circulatory, respiratory, and gastrointestinal disease; to infant mortality; and to arthritis. Infections also complicate a wide range of injuries and have been found to cause some malignancies (Haggett, 1994). However, US death rates over the course of the twentieth century demonstrate that mortality had been declining steadily, except for one upturn in the 1918–19 influenza epidemic. Although by the end of the 1970s, the longest-lived survivors were not living very much longer than they were in the seventeenth century, premature death had been largely excluded from human experience in the developed world. The risks of dying in infancy, childhood and young adulthood had fallen dramatically, and the risk of dying in later years fallen by about half. By the late 1970s, the developing world pattern was that a small percentage of newborns died in their first year, but then only a tiny number died in successive years, until about the 70th year of life, after which the risk of death grew rapidly with each succeeding year. Continuing a pattern that began in the mid-1800s, gathered force after the discovery of bacteria, and advanced rapidly after the Second World War, by the 1970s death in the developed world was confined for the most part to the elderly (Urquhart & Heilmann, 1984).

At the beginning of the twentieth century, infectious diseases were the main killers, but by 1940 TB, nephritis, diphtheria, and 'diarrhoea, enteritis and ulceration of the intestines' had disappeared from the top ten US causes of death, while deaths from heart disease increased sharply, as did to a lesser extent deaths from cancer due to smoking. By 1940 heart disease and cancer were already in first and second place. Suicide first appeared in the top ten in 1979, not because there were more suicides, but because of other causes of death had fallen. By the late 1970s, the leading causes of death, once dominated by infectious disease, were dominated by chronic diseases and cancer (Urquhart & Heilmann, 1984).

The concern in the late 1970s was not that infectious diseases might make a reappearance, but that the successes of biomedicine against infectious diseases would lead to a population crisis. A decade later, Ebola, Legionnaires' disease and other infections newly discovered or rising in prevalence through the 1970s would retrospectively be classified

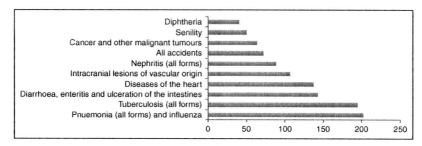

Figure 2.1 Ten leading causes of death – death rates US per 100,000 1900

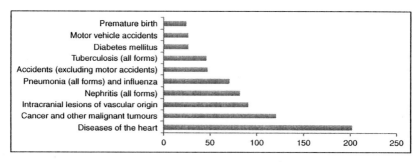

Figure 2.2 Ten leading causes of death – death rates US per 100,000 1940

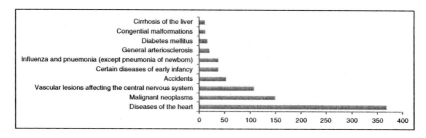

Figure 2.3 Ten leading causes of death – death rates US per 100,000 1960

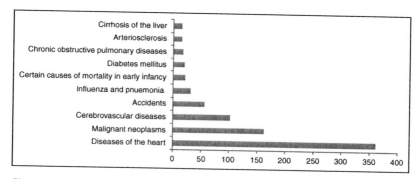

Figure 2.4   Ten leading causes of death – death rates US per 100,000 1970

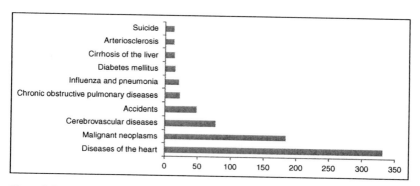

Figure 2.5   Ten leading causes of death – death rates US per 100,000 1979
Source: All data for Figures 2.1–2.5 from Urquhart & Heilmann, 1984.

as 'emerging or re-emerging'. From the perspective of 1981, however, infectious diseases were, if not conquered, then at least not a pressing concern.

No ambitious young doctor or research scientist would have been interested in a career in the backwaters of infectious diseases. Most medical and scientific funding bodies were awarding very few grants for research into infectious diseases. For example, by 1978, roughly half of all research proposals submitted to the NIH were for research into cancer (Chubin & Studer, 1978). Medical students were advised to avoid specialising in infectious disease because it was a dying field (Lewontin & Levins, 2003). By 1980, nearly all deaths in developed countries were due to cardiovascular diseases, cancer, accidents, chronic diseases and suicides. As a result, governments across the developed world dismantled or neglected their now apparently redundant public health infrastructure.

And while attention was firmly focused elsewhere, along came, as the musician Prince put it, 'a big disease with a little name'.

3
AIDS and the End of the Golden Age of Medicine

The appearance of AIDS in 1981 marks not only a critical shift in the atmosphere of optimism surrounding the 'conquest' of infectious diseases, but also a break with the previous history of medicine. Historians of medicine tend to locate AIDS as the latest in a long line of plagues. Yet the AIDS pandemic was, and still is, different: perhaps as much a socio-cultural and political phenomenon as a medical one. Arguably, any new infectious disease that happened to appear at that juncture in history would have created a media storm greater than did those infectious diseases of just a few years earlier. However, the AIDS epidemic's heady cocktail of sex, drugs, race, religion and politics created a societal and media event that would irrevocably alter the cultural landscape.

Although early speculation about the source of the HIV virus being a zoonotic disease of African green monkeys has since been discredited (see below), it is now generally accepted on the basis of genetic evidence that the source of the two strains of HIV – HIV-1 and HIV-2 – are from similar simian (monkey or ape) immunodeficiency viruses (SIV) found in chimpanzees (SIVcpz) and sooty mangabeys (SIVsm) respectively (Hillis, 2000). Further evidence for such a link comes from the geographical coincidence between the natural habitat of the sooty mangabeys and HIV-2 in coastal West Africa; and from the fact that SIVsm and HIV-2 virus derived from animals and humans from the same geographic area were found to be closely related, which implicates hunting as a route of transmission. Although not as clear-cut, the evidence for the origins of HIV-1 points to SIVcpz transmission from chimpanzees to humans in West equatorial Africa, where chimpanzees have been found infected with genetically closely related viruses (Hahn & Shaw, 2000).

Although there is no evidence for how the virus jumped species to humans, it has been hypothesised that both SIVcpz and SIVsm were probably transmitted to humans as a result of biting or exposure to infected animal blood as a result of hunting, butchering or consumption of infected wild animals for food, so-called 'bushmeat'. There is also direct evidence for HIV-1 infection from SIVsm by direct blood and virus contact in health care and primate centre workers (Hahn & Shaw, 2000). It has therefore also been hypothesised that the jump from monkeys to humans may have been facilitated by the sharp increase in the trade in monkeys to the West in the 1960s for medical research, which would have entailed extensive handling and close contact with captured animals both in Africa and in the West (Myers et al., 1992). Although it has been suggested that transmission could have occurred via poliovirus cultured in chimpanzee kidney cells in Central Africa between 1957 and 1960, this is generally considered unlikely. On the basis of molecular analyses of the different strains of HIV and SIV, it is now generally accepted that the HIV virus was transmitted to humans on numerous occasions between 1915 and 1941. The most widely accepted hypothesis is that the virus was transmitted to humans at some point in the 1800s or early 1900s but remained isolated until about 1930, when the virus began to spread through different human populations and to diversify (Hillis, 2000).

When doctors encounter unusual and unexplained cases of diseases, they publish reports of them in medical journals so that similar rare cases can be identified elsewhere and links made between them. A search of the literature for sporadic cases suggestive of AIDS between 1950 and 1980 revealed 19 reported cases from North America, Western Europe, Africa and the Middle East. The first case of what would later become known as AIDS was published in the medical literature in 1953, although that diagnosis would only be confirmed retrospectively. AIDS is therefore probably an old disease, but one that went unrecognised because of its sporadic occurrence (Huminer et al., 1987). Retrospective testing for HIV antibodies of sera collected in the 1970s in association with hepatitis B studies in San Francisco, Los Angeles and New York suggests that HIV-1 entered the US population sometime in the middle of the 1970s (Myers et al., 1992).

Early reporting of AIDS

Sporadic case reports in medical journals would not have alerted the attention of epidemiologists at the time they were published. For that to happen, a cluster of cases with a similar clinical picture would have to appear in the same time or place. That cluster was first reported on 5 June 1981, when the US Morbidity and Mortality Report (CDC, 1981) described of a group of young men with *Pneumocystis carinii* pneumonia (a rare type of pneumonia usually only seen in patients with severe immunodeficiency associated with other serious illness) and Kaposi's sarcoma (a skin cancer usually only seen in elderly men of Mediterranean origin). This group of patients was also suffering from widespread immunodeficiency, apparently without reason. The only thing that seemed to link them was that they were all homosexual men. In response to the report of this cluster, the CDC started a nation-wide surveillance programme the following month. In December of 1981, these cases were reported in the *New England Journal of Medicine* in greater detail, including what was to become recognised as the hallmark deficiency in the CD4 T-cells (Gottlieb et al., 1981).

Epidemiological evidence pointed to a sexually transmitted infectious cause from the outset, yet the new disease was originally dubbed 'gay cancer', perhaps reflecting the *zeitgeist* of the time, when cancer was thought to be more serious than infectious diseases. The 'gay cancer' label was soon changed to Gay Related Immune Deficiency (GRID), and in September 1982 the CDC announced creation of the official acronym, Acquired Immune Deficiency Syndrome (AIDS).

The *Los Angeles Times* and the *San Francisco Chronicle* both ran short reports of the new illness within days of the original CDC report; the *New York Times* of 3 July 1981, on page 20, printed an article head-lined 'Rare cancer seen in 41 homosexuals'. The *New York Native* of 27 July ran an article headlined 'Cancer in the Gay Community' (Mass, 2004). Yet apart from this initial tiny amount of coverage, for many months the early reports of AIDS were otherwise ignored by the mass media on both sides of the Atlantic. Almost a year later, on 31 May 1982, by which point a new case of AIDS was being reported every day, the *Los Angeles Times* ran a front-page piece entitled 'Mysterious Fever Now an Epidemic'. It was not until June 1982 that the US TV network news first covered the story (Treichler, 1999). The gay com-munity in NYC were particularly bitter about coverage of AIDS in the *New York Times*, which only ran seven articles on AIDS in the first 18 months of the epidemic, compared with 54 articles over three months of a scare involving poisoned Tylenol (paracetamol) in 1982, which had a far lower death toll (Altman, 1986). Early reports of the AIDS epidemic were similarly ignored in Britain (Watney, 1987) and France (Herzlich & Pierret, 1989).

It thus took many months, years even, before the implications of this new epidemic penetrated the collective consciousness. The AIDS epidemic contradicted the prevailing paradigm that infectious diseases were 'a thing of the past'. One reason why AIDS was not accepted as a serious public health threat in the early years of the epidemic may well have been *because* it was an infectious disease (Berkelman & Freeman, 2004). Another difficulty in raising media interest related to who was affected. Media editors refused to see how a story about the health of homosexuals and drug users could interest their readers, who were assumed to be a homogenous audience of (white) heterosexual non-drug users. Editors felt that AIDS failed that test of newsworthiness, whereas other diseases such as Legionnaires' disease or toxic shock syndrome, which threatened people like them, passed. This angle was taken as common-sense in newsrooms (Allen, 2002).

The initial response, or lack of it, to AIDS from the media was mirrored at a political level. In Britain, Mrs Thatcher's Conservative government ignored the subject entirely until 1985. In the USA, AIDS gained far less attention from President Reagan than the threatened epidemic of swine fever had from President Ford in 1976 (Altman, 1986). Indeed, US federal officials were openly antipathetic to gay men and drug users and deliberately blocked attempts to respond to the AIDS crisis. For example, the Surgeon General C. Everett Koop later complained that he was not allowed to speak about AIDS publicly until President Reagan's second term in 1985. Whenever Koop spoke on a health issue at a press conference or on a network morning TV show, the government public affairs people told the media in advance that he would not answer questions on AIDS, and was not to be asked any questions on the subject (Lederberg et al., 1992).

High-risk groups

The epidemic only really began to attract media coverage from about 1983. At this stage, two aspects of the new disease were still a mystery: The first was what was causing it. Several theories were proposed, although from the outset a viral cause was suspected. This was confirmed in May 1983, when Dr Luc Montagnier at the Pasteur Institute in Paris discovered the virus that caused AIDS, which he called *Lymphadenopathy associated virus* (LAV). Dr Robert Gallo at the US National Cancer Institute claimed the discovery as his own, and called it HTLVIII. The discovery of the viral cause of AIDS was announced the following year. Later, the term human immunodeficiency virus (HIV) was coined. Once a viral cause for the syndrome had been established, a means to test for the presence of antibodies to the virus could be developed. In 1985 the test capable of detecting HIV antibodies in the blood became widely available.

The second mystery at this point was why the disease seemed to be affecting only members of certain groups. The CDC specified certain 'sub-groups' 'at risk for AIDS'. These were: (1) male homosexuals or bisexual men and their sexual contacts; (2) female and heterosexual male intravenous drug users; (3) male homosexuals or bisexuals who were intravenous drug users; (4) people with haemophilia or another blood coagulation disorder; and (5) heterosexual contacts of those at increased risk. In late 1982, acknowledging the high incidence of the syndrome in people from Haiti, Haitians were added to those considered at risk (the CDC eventually withdrew the classification of Haitians as 'high risk' in 1985).

This classification of what became known as the 4H 'at risk' groups – homosexuals, heroin addicts, haemophiliacs and Haitians – soon became popularly recast as 'HIV risk groups'. One unintended consequence of the notion of 'risk groups' was that all gay men, intravenous drug users and Haitians became identified as members of a risk group, whether or not they engaged in risky behaviour. The use of these categories to characterise who was 'at risk' diverted attention from everyone else, who became grouped together as 'the general population' and who were thought *not* to be at risk (Schiller et al., 1994). The notion of 'high risk' groups was used to mask prejudice, particularly against gay men, excluding them from life insurance, employment, legal safeguards and so on.

Faced with the devastation that the epidemic was causing, the gay community itself organised initiatives from the early 1980s to raise awareness of AIDS and promote what by 1983 had become known as 'safer sex' amongst gay men. Highly politicised groups were set up, the first of which, Gay Men's Health Crisis, in New York, became the model for similar groups elsewhere, including the Terrence Higgins Trust in the UK. These groups campaigned to lobby politicians for resources, both for treatment and for research. Changes in the sexual behaviour of gay men soon became apparent throughout the Western world, well before governments belatedly ran AIDS prevention campaigns. As a result of this community action, there was a sharp decline not only in the numbers of gay men reported as engaging in high-risk sexual activities, but also correspondingly in the numbers of new HIV infections of gay men (King, 1993).

The gay plague

The identification of AIDS with gay men, and to a lesser extent with drug users, led to the disease and its sufferers being largely ignored and neglected by governments and the mainstream media. AIDS was cast as an exclusively gay disease: the 'gay plague'. Although there was evidence from the outset that there might be modes of transmission other than through anal sex (between men), the idea that AIDS could be transmitted through heterosexual sex was resisted or denied; and while AIDS affected only those in 'high-risk groups', it remained of little interest to the media and did not capture the imagination of the public. Furthermore, the epidemiological term 'high-risk group', particularly as applied to gay men, was understood to mean not that gay men *were vulnerable to* contracting HIV, but that *they posed a risk* to other people (Watney, 1989).

The use of the plague metaphor in the context of AIDS has a number of dimensions that bear unpacking. Plagues usually come from somewhere else, from foreigners, from people other than *us*. The first 'work' that the plague metaphor does is to set up a dichotomy between *us* and *them*. On the one hand *others* pose a threat to *people like us*, and on the other hand *they* are so different from *us* that any perceived risk is simultaneously distanced and contained. Vocabulary used to describe people in HIV risk groups made them seem exotic and separate from the mainstream. For example, households of gay men were never described as families, and even in the social scientific and medical literature, lifetime partners were described as 'sexual contacts' rather than spouses, partners or lovers. Neither drug users nor gay men were ever described in terms of their biological families – as mothers, fathers, children, siblings – apart from in cases where children had been infected by their mothers (Schiller et al., 1994). This placing of gay men outside of, and threatening to, 'family values' was later institutionalised in the UK with the notorious Clause 28 of The Local Government Act 1988, which forbade local authorities from promoting homosexuality as a 'pretended family relationship'.

Sex between men was automatically framed as promiscuous, and redefined as medically unsafe. The idea that the 'gay plague' would 'leak out' from 'high-risk groups' into 'the general population' became a media obsession. Both the popular and serious press of the period constantly referred to its readers as if they could not possibly identify with the vast majority of those most closely affected by the illness: gay men. News reports about AIDS consistently focused on the 'threat' that gay and bisexual men posed to 'the general population' and refused to allow any identification *with* gay men under any circumstances. The gay man became 'he-with-whom-identification-is-forbidden' (Watney, 1987).

The association between AIDS and homosexuality fell on particularly fertile ground among the newly politicised religious right, particularly in the USA, where the AIDS epidemic coincided with the growing political clout of the so-called 'Moral Majority'. They saw traditional values under siege, and were anxious about the sexual freedoms of the 1960s and 1970s, which they felt had led to AIDS.

The 'gay plague' metaphor thus meshed with fundamentalist Christian beliefs that homosexuality itself was a sin, and into the religious horror of anal sex. As AIDS transmission was characterised as being exclusively through anal sex, many commentators suggested that the virus actually originated in and from the anus. AIDS thus became the metaphor for the sin of homosexuality, and more generally for the sin of all sexual pleasure. The culprit was homosexual anal sex, and by extension gay men themselves, and like the Biblical plagues of Egypt, the punishment for their sin was disease and death (Poirier, 1988).

In Britain, homophobic bishops became a tabloid staple of AIDS reporting, yet the political influence of the religious right was never as powerful in the more secular (northern) European countries as it was in the USA. French newspapers of the period emphasised that the punitive 'divine punishment' interpretation had, like AIDS itself, developed in the USA – they related it to 'Anglo-Saxon Puritanism', to 'Reaganism' or to the US 'Moral Majority' movement (Herzlich & Pierret, 1989).

Long before Freud, medical discourse had treated homosexuality as a disease. HIV, like homosexuality, was said to be latent, in people who may not know they have it, and ready to corrupt and betray the carrier. AIDS was thus elided with the notion of homosexuality as a disease and both were said to threaten the survival of the human race. Many said, sometimes quite directly, that the need to eradicate homosexuality and homosexuals took precedence over the need to eradicate the disease. The promotion of condom use was rejected by the religious right as condoning a sexual practice prohibited in the Bible. In 1987, by a vote of 98 to two, the US Senate approved the notorious 'Helms Amendment', introduced by Senator Jesse Helms, which prohibited federal funding to any organisation, including Gay Men's Health Crisis, that 'promoted homosexuality', interpreted as including any gay-positive material counselling safer sex. (The Helms Amendment was legally challenged and overturned in 1992.)

Routine close contact

In May 1983 the first big spike of media interest in AIDS was prompted by a paper published in the *Journal of the American Medical Association* (Oleske et al., 1983). It described eight children (of whom four had died) from the New Jersey area, who were born into families with recognised risk factors for AIDS, and had suffered from recurrent illnesses and failure to thrive. The authors suggested that sexual contact, drug use, or exposure to blood products were not necessary for the disease to be transmitted. In it, they wrote '[T]he epidemiology of AIDS may now have taken an ominous new turn . . . It seems more plausible to us that the illnesses in these youngsters were related in some way to household exposure and their residence in communities involved in the current epidemic of AIDS' (Oleske et al., 1983: 2345–8). Thus the paper prompted the proposition that HIV might be transmissible to the entire population through 'routine close contact'.

At this point, it was still being denied that HIV could be transmitted via heterosexual sex. One of the major turning points in raising the public(s) consciousness about heterosexual AIDS was the announcement that the Hollywood actor Rock Hudson had AIDS in June 1985 and his subsequent death in October of that year. Hudson's announcement resulted in the number of newspaper articles published on the subject of AIDS soaring by 500 per cent (Gardner, 2008) and prompted President Reagan's first acknowledgement of the epidemic in September of that year. Ironically, given Hudson's previously unacknowledged homosexuality, his death marked the point at which AIDS ceased to be seen strictly as a gay disease. Hudson prompted audience identification with the human interest aspect of AIDS, something that had clearly proved difficult with gay men and others affected by the disease, and points to the way in which Western celebrity culture provides a sense of shared experience with 'stars'. While homosexuality and drug use were distant from the experience of many, people felt that they somehow knew Hudson personally and had something in common with him (Treichler, 1999).

Hudson's fate was to join those other gay men with AIDS who had come to visually represent the epidemic – the 'face of AIDS'. 'Before' and 'after' pictures of 'AIDS victims' became a macabre journalistic cliché. Sadistic images of gay men with bodies 'all but stripped of the sensual luxury of flesh, and . . . faces . . . blistered and swollen beyond human recognition' became the authentic cadaver of Oscar Wilde's *Picture of Dorian Gray*, 'wrinkled, withered and loathsome of visage' (Watney, 1994: 30). The jutting bones, sunken glassy eyes and listless expressions of despair were so ubiquitous in the media coverage that journalists reportedly rejected photographing healthier-looking 'specimens' because they did not 'look the part'. These 'before' and 'after' photographs were often accompanied by textual references to gay or bisexual men who, like Hudson, had become 'unmasked' by AIDS, who could no longer pretend to be 'one of us'. Their exposure as pariahs again fed into religious notions of sin and suffering as a punishment for their previous 'self-indulgent lifestyle' (not lives). Their suffering was thus subtly signalled as their 'just deserts', from which neither their fame nor wealth could protect them (Kitzinger, 1995). The message was clear: Homosexuality = AIDS = death.

The collective scapegoating of gay men was often focused on individual apparently vengeful or irresponsible 'AIDS carriers'. The most infamous of these was a Canadian air steward, Gaetan Dugas, who epidemiologists established had had sexual links with at least 40 of the first 248 gay men diagnosed with AIDS in the USA. For Americans, Dugas personified the culpable foreigner who had covertly transported HIV into the USA, exposing the increased permeability of national borders and the vulnerability of American citizens (King, 2003b).

In his history of the early AIDS epidemic, *And the Band Played On*, Randy Shilts (1987) demonises Dugas – controversially dubbed *patient zero* – with language that evokes both a modern day Typhoid Mary and the evil queen from Snow White (Williamson, 1989): 'Gaeten examined himself in the mirror...a few more spots had the temerity to appear on his face...he smiled at the thought, "I'm still the prettiest one"'. While Shilts' book blames the entire governmental system for failing to respond to the AIDS crisis, he nevertheless cannot entirely resist the wish for a source of contamination to be found and blamed. For Shilts, *patient zero* epitomises those gay man who behaved less than sensibly in the early days of the epidemic, and by locating blame in a single individual he inverts, but does not challenge, the wider tendency to blame all gay men for AIDS (Watney, 1994).

Heterosexual AIDS

Despite the accumulating medical evidence, even as late as the end of 1985 the media on both sides of the Atlantic remained convinced that AIDS was not a threat to heterosexuals. Anal sex, particularly receptive anal sex, was said to be the unique danger for contracting HIV, because the anus 'wasn't designed for sex' and could tear during penetration. Vaginas, on the other hand, were designed 'by nature' to accommodate a penis and for childbirth, a mindset that has been dubbed the 'vulnerable anus and rugged vagina' thesis (Treichler, 1999).

Although there were no dramatic discoveries in 1986, by the end of that year the major US news magazines were running cover stories about how AIDS could pose a danger to heterosexuals. Then, in late 1986, the CDC reclassified a significant number of previously 'unexplained' AIDS cases, and acknowledged that they had been heterosexually transmitted. Subsequently, the US National Academy of Sciences and the IOM issued a report warning that HIV could be transmissible to and from women and men. The US Surgeon General held a press conference to announce that he viewed AIDS as a potential threat to every sexually active person and advocating the institution of immediate explicit sex education. In January 1987, the cover story of the *US News and World Report* headline read: 'Suddenly, the disease of *them* is the disease of *us*', with the 'us' illustrated by a picture of a young, white, urban professional man and woman (Triechler, 1988).

In the later years of the 1980s, in light of the by then incontrovertible evidence of heterosexual transmission of HIV, governments around the world launched politically sensitive public education campaigns. These campaigns were often characterised by interdepartmental and inter-professional conflicts, and by conflicts with AIDS activists. In the UK for example, the 1986 campaign of Mrs Thatcher's conservative govern-ment featured tombstones engraved with the message: 'AIDS – Don't die of ignorance'. The subtext was moral rather than medical: the message was reduce the numbers of sexual partners, and if you did have sex with someone you did not know (or trust), then to use a condom. This mes-sage – choose carefully *or* use a condom – was at odds with the franker and more 'sex positive' message favoured by AIDS activists: which was to enjoy sex, explore other, non-penetrative forms of eroticism, and when you do have penetrative sex, always use a condom, whether or not you know your own or your partner's HIV status. The government message was aimed at heterosexuals – 'the general population' – who were choos-ing sexual partners from a population with a very low prevalence of HIV. Yet AIDS activists argued that for those choosing sexual partners from a population with a high HIV prevalence – namely gay men – the message *not* to use a condom every time was a potentially very dangerous one.

1986 also saw Australia's first government AIDS campaign. Australian television advertisements showed the image of a 'grim reaper' who bowled a number of 'ordinary' people down in a bowling alley. This 'AIDS equals death' message carried with it older associations of the 'grim reaper' accompanying famine, plague and divine retribution.

In both the Australian grim reaper campaign, and the UK 'Don't die of ignorance' one, the message was clear: what had up to that point been a 'gay plague' was now a 'plague' that threatened all members of society (Lupton, 1994).

One view that ran counter to the prevailing liberal/medical orthodoxy was that of the so-called 'AIDS dissidents'. The most prominent of these was Peter Duesberg, a Professor of molecular biology at the University of California who in 1987 argued that infection with the HIV retrovirus was incidental to AIDS. Together with other proponents of the view that HIV did not cause AIDS, Duesberg argued that AIDS was caused by personal behaviour, notably recreational (non-injecting) drug use, or (later) by the medicines used to treat AIDS patients.

The 'AIDS dissidents' claims were debated in scientific journals and repeatedly refuted, even by a specialist panel assembled by the National Academy of Sciences. For example, evidence from studies showed no difference in the prevalence of AIDS between gay men who had or gay men who had not used recreational drugs. Claims that AIDS in haemophiliacs was as a result of haemophilia itself being immunosuppressive were undermined by studies demonstrating that haemophiliacs who had never received blood products showed no evidence of AIDS. However, the dissidents' arguments continued to be reported by the press as evidence of some sort of 'homosexual conspiracy' propagated by the 'AIDS industry'. The success of Highly Active Anti-retroviral Therapy (HAART) in the late 1990s led to a dramatic fall in illness and death rates in those who were able to receive it. HAART was predicated on reducing the viral load of HIV. This effectively undermined Duesberg's position and left little room to doubt that HIV is the driving factor in AIDS (Delaney, 2000).

The framing of AIDS as a 'gay plague' up to 1986 had served to distance the threat that the disease could pose to the 'general population'. In the final years of that decade the emphasis changed dramatically, away from AIDS as a gay disease and towards the threat that the epidemic posed to heterosexuals. The media coverage of AIDS in this period was characterised by several dominant archetypes. First were the 'guilty' victims: gay men, drug users and 'prostitutes' punished for their deviant activities. The antithesis of this archetype was the 'innocent' victim, often represented by white, married, middle-class heterosexual women, unknowingly, maliciously or carelessly infected by their duplicitous 'AIDS carrier' partners, who were later exposed as bisexual or having a history of drug use. Haemophiliacs were also cast as 'innocent' victims, but the most 'innocent' victims of all were children, 'blamelessly' infected through blood transfusions or by their deviant mothers (Lupton, 1999a).

While the threat of HIV transmission through unprotected sex was downplayed or ignored, the 'innocent victim' narrative was routinely presented in the media as being typical of cases of HIV transmission. One variant of this, which clearly had great cultural resonance, was the careless or malicious 'AIDS carrier' story. Respondents in focus groups spontaneously exchanged stories of a man or woman leaving the message 'Welcome to the AIDS club' scrawled in lipstick on a mirror following a one-night stand. This urban myth was recounted as a real event that actually happened to a friend of a friend (Eldridge et al., 1997).

Another variant of the AIDS carrier/innocent victim narrative played out in the USA, where six patients of the same Florida dentist developed HIV. The dentist in question, David Acer, was a gay man who later died of AIDS. Most famous of his patients was 23-year-old Kimberley Bergalis, who publically proclaimed she was a virgin and that therefore the only way she could have been infected was by Acer. Bergalis' undoubtedly tragic story was used by those who campaigned for mandatory HIV testing as a form of HIV prevention. Press coverage of the story offered up a series of double messages, on the one hand warning against exaggerated fears and of the ethical and practical problems surrounding mandatory testing, while simultaneously featuring screaming headlines clearly designed to pander to exactly those fears and foster the sense of crisis that added fuel to fire of the those who called for mandatory testing (Park, 1993). A CDC investigation later concluded that Acer *had* infected his patients, making it the only known case of health-care-worker to patient HIV transmission. However, in 1994 a CBS television *60 Minutes* documentary questioned the CDC conclusions, revealing the previously undisclosed information that Bergalis lied about her sexual experience and had a disease that could have been sexually transmitted (Brown, 1996).

Over the next couple of years, the media interest in AIDS diminished, although there was a storm of controversy in 1988 following publication of *Crisis: Heterosexual Behavior in the Age of AIDS,* by the famous sex researchers Masters and Johnson. In it they argued ' ... categorically that infection with the AIDS virus [*sic*] does *not* require intimate sexual contact or sharing intravenous needles: transmission can, and does, occur as a result of person-to-person contact in which blood or other body fluids from a person who is harbouring the virus are splashed onto or rubbed against someone else, even if this is a single, isolated occurrence' (Masters et al., 1988: 2).

Like so much written on AIDS at the time, Masters and Johnson's book focused on the handful of cases where HIV seemed to have been transmitted by means other than unprotected sex, such as the three health-care workers who had apparently been infected with HIV from contact with blood but without needle-stick injury (CDC, 1987). With these extremely rare and unexplained cases as a starting point, they extrapolate a series of fantasies of the dangers lurking in participation in sport, in sitting on toilet seats and so on: 'Is it possible to become infected with the AIDS virus [sic] in a touch football game, on the soccer field, while sliding into second base, or on the basketball court? In a word, yes.' ... 'Can you catch AIDS [sic] from a toilet seat?' '...if infected blood (from a cut, scrape, ulcer, blister, or rash on the buttocks) or infected semen (either dripped from the penis or spilled from a condom) is inadvertently left on a toilet seat and someone who comes in contact with this material also happens to have a break in the skin at the point of contact, the virus may enter the body and infection may occur' (Masters et al., 1988: 32–93).

African AIDS

While Masters and Johnson were playing on *deep-seated* American fantasy fears of contaminated toilets – fears that can be traced back to the pre-First World War anti-syphilis campaigns (Brandt, 1985) – it was becoming clear that in Africa, AIDS was an all-too-real disaster. By the end of 1981, doctors in the Zairian capital of Kinshasa had also begun to notice patients with similar symptoms to those reported in America and whose immune systems seemed to be collapsing (Lamey & Malemeka, 1982). As it became increasingly clear that a parallel AIDS epidemic was unfolding in Africa, Western doctors and scientists became obsessed with discovering the African origin of AIDS.

In 1985, a 'Conference on African AIDS' was held in Brussels. US scientists reported that over half of African blood samples stored from the 1960s and 1970s were infected with HIV. This seemed to confirm that AIDS was an African disease that had been present for centuries in Central Africa. However, the type of test the US scientists used had produced false positive results. Other (Western) scientists who replicated the testing found only two per cent HIV prevalence in the same stored blood samples. The latter result was announced in June 1985 but failed to attract the same media attention as the initial incorrect conclusions. African doctors found the implication that AIDS has been present and unnoticed in Africa for a long time insulting (Sabatier, 1988).

The Brussels conference and these false results caused much resentment in Africa and amongst African doctors and researchers who had not been consulted, and who objected to the implication that AIDS was an 'old' African disease. One immediate after-effect of the conference was the adoption of secrecy by African health authorities, who might otherwise have approached AIDS differently. Across Europe, in India, in the Soviet Union and elsewhere, AIDS was often blamed on African students. In 1987, Belgium started to introduce compulsory HIV tests for foreign students on government grants – all of whom were African. In the same year India began testing all foreign students, 85 per cent of whom were African (Sabatier, 1988).

As the notion that AIDS was 'an old disease of Africa' and had been 'lurking' in some imaginary 'isolated tribe' became increasingly untenable, attention moved to a more recent monkey origin for HIV. Early speculation about the simian origin of HIV was based on genetic analysis of viruses isolated from green monkeys and humans in West Africa, and from macaque monkeys in US laboratories. African green monkeys are known to act as a reservoir for yellow fever and Marburg disease. A simian origin for AIDS was hypothesised after Harvard scientists claimed in 1985 to have isolated a virus that was closely related to HIV – STLV-3agm – from green monkeys caught in the wild in Africa (Kanki et al., 1985).

African commentators objected to this green monkey theory on that grounds that it 'cohabit[ed] easily with racist notions that Africans are evolutionarily closer to sub-human primates, or with images gleaned from Tarzan movies of Africans living in trees like monkeys' (Chirimuuta & Chirimuuta, 1987: 71). In early 1988, Kanki and Essex, the Harvard scientists behind the green monkey theory, partly retracted their theory and announced that contamination must have occurred and that their viruses had in fact not come from West Africa but from captive monkeys (Sabatier, 1988).

Partly as a result of these types of (Western) scientific 'conclusions' about the African origin of AIDS, Africans subsequently doubted all Western AIDS science. African doctors questioned the numbers of diagnoses of AIDS in Africa, particularly where HIV testing was not carried out, or where a positive result was not confirmed by another different type of test for the virus, as would have happened in the West. They also suggested that the signs and symptoms of 'AIDS' may have been confused with other diseases common in the tropics by Western doctors unfamiliar with tropical diseases. They dismissed the argument made that the lack of diagnostic facilities in Africa had led to AIDS first being identified in the USA rather than in Africa, pointing out that there was a well-documented increase in opportunistic infections in teaching hospitals in sub-Saharan Africa *after* the onset of the US epidemic. Africans, not unreasonably, suggested that the reason that the epidemic was first recognised in the USA and in Europe was because that was where it originated. They suggested that, as was the case in Haiti, HIV was then spread to Africans through Westerners' sexual exploitation of the locals. Africans argued that racist associations of black people with dirt, disease and excessive sexuality influenced researchers to over-diagnose AIDS in black people or identify them as its source (Chirimuuta & Chirimuuta, 1987).

AIDS appeared at roughly the same time in the USA, Europe, Africa and Haiti, and given that all societies had different social structures that facilitated its spread in different ways, there seems little to be gained in pointing a finger of blame in any direction. Social changes in the West in the 1960s and 1970s, such as the sexual revolution and the rise of injecting drug use, led to Western epidemics of HIV/AIDS. In Africa different social changes were instrumental in fanning the epidemic. Those changes related to the end of colonial rule in Africa, one legacy of which was the growth of large cities as poverty forced widespread migration from rural to urban areas, and the consequent breakdown of traditional family and social structures. Poverty and racist housing policies forced men to move away from their homes and wives for long periods to find work in towns and mines, and poverty made selling or exchanging sex a necessity for some women. For others, the end of colonialism meant the increased opportunity for legal and illegal travel to and from the developing world. The widespread introduction of vaccination programmes, with the deliberate or inadvertent reuse of needles, also led to HIV infections in some cases (Hahn & Shaw, 2000; Hillis, 2000).

If African AIDS was problematic for Africans, then it was equally problematic for Western scientists and epidemiologists, because it contradicted the prevailing Western notion that AIDS was a gay disease and that the unique risk for HIV transmission was anal sex between men. The 'cultural explanations' of the 1:1 AIDS ratio of men to women in Africa and Haiti included a range of exotica, including: African promiscuity; widespread prevalence of disease and or malnutrition; anal intercourse as a method of birth control; various rituals, voodoo or practices of 'native healers' or 'witch doctors'; female circumcision; lack of circumcision in men; violent (dry) sex; ritual scarification; quasi-homosexual transmission (from a previous lover's semen left in the vagina); bestiality; even cannibalism (Treichler, 1999; Watney,

1994). It seemed inconceivable that the African AIDS epidemic could be the result of unremarkable unprotected heterosexual sex.

The tropes used to explain African AIDS fed on older colonial notions of Africa as the 'dark continent', disease- and disaster-ridden, as imagined in Joseph Conrad's *Heart of Darkness*. One key colonialist trope was 'animalisation'. This notion was rooted in religious and philosophical traditions which drew sharp boundaries between humans and animals, and in which 'the civilised' suppressed all animal-like characteristics of the self. Colonialist/racist discourse renders colonised people as bestial 'savages and wild animals'. Africa and Africans in particular are projected as childlike, as evidenced in the racist habit of calling adult colonised men 'boy'; or as hyper-masculine and hypersexual. (Asia by contrast is projected as dreamy, submissive and feminine.) In racist colonial hierarchies, the colonised also tend to be viewed as vegetative and instinctual rather than learned and cultural (Shohat & Stam, 1994).

In the discourse around HIV, countless anecdotes concerning 'dirty' hospitals, 'out-of-date' medical equipment, sharing of syringes and so on positioned 'primitive' African hospitals in relation to the more advanced and civilised West. The implication was that 'African AIDS' could be explained away as a product of African medicine. Black Africans were depicted, like Africa itself, as dying slowly, listless, diseased, starving, as if AIDS were a disease of 'African-ness', the viral embodiment of the continent (Watney, 1994).

For their part, Africans also constructed AIDS in terms of their colonial histories, but from an African perspective, AIDS mapped on to postcolonial discourses of the history of the exploitation of the continent. African conspiracy theories blamed Western science for HIV; specifically it was claimed that AIDS was the product of US military germ warfare experiments. Another reaction from Africa and elsewhere (China, India, Japan, Malaysia, the Philippines, Mexico, Venezuela and the USSR) was to blame AIDS on Westerners' degenerate sexual habits. 'Ex-pats' and tourists were accused of 'spreading' HIV, exporting a culture of pornography and easy sex. Africans regarded the promotion of condom use with suspicion, as birth control is frequently regarded by black Africans as a facet of white genocidal aspirations. In pre-independence Rhodesia (Zimbabwe) for example, family planning was opposed by both the main African nationalist parties (Sabatier, 1988).

As well as blaming Westerners for AIDS, Africans also sometimes blamed ethnic minorities within their own countries, such as Indian doctors; or they blamed neighbouring countries for the problem. Uganda blamed Kenya and vice versa for example (Sabatier, 1988).

The African response inverted the (Western) worldview, which linked AIDS to Africa. As with the scapegoating of gay men in the West, Africans located the responsibility for and threat of AIDS externally. African conspiracy theories about AIDS make sense in the context of a continent that was so brutally exploited by colonialism, and later by global capitalism. Many Africans connected AIDS with the covert apartheid era biological weapons programme – Project Coast – intended for the assassination of state enemies within and outside the country, with unethical pharmaceutical research carried out in Africa (Goldacre, 2008), or with the environmental recklessness of multinational corporations in these countries.

The Soviet Union also blamed AIDS on a US conspiracy. In 1985 an article in *Literaturnaya Gazeta*, the official journal of the Soviet Writers' Union, entitled *Panic in the West, or What Lies behind the Sensationalism of AIDS*, argued that AIDS was made by biological warriors at Fort Detrick, Maryland, in conjunction with CDC scientists (Nelkin & Gilman, 1988). Like all conspiracy theories and urban myths about AIDS, the notion that AIDS is an American or Western invention reveals a way of making sense of the epidemic that resonates with the individual fears and collective histories either of colonialism or Cold War politics.

The 'degaying' of AIDS

By the end of the 1980s in most Western countries, there had been a change in the accepted orthodoxy about 'high-risk groups'. There was a widespread feeling that it was a historical accident that AIDS had 'landed' first amongst gay men. Preparations were made for what was felt would be the inevitable next stage of the epidemic in the 'general population'.

Given the apparent success of community-based initiatives amongst gay men in adopting safer sex, it was felt that the 'battle had been won' as regards health promotion for gay men and safer sex. Levels of comfort with discussions of gay sex amongst many biomedical scientists and the conservative administrations on both sides of the Atlantic ranged from squeamishness to outright homophobia. The combination of these factors led to a situation where government health education resources were targeted at 'the general population' (heterosexuals) and were rarely addressed to the group who, at that time, constituted over 80 per cent of Western AIDS cases. The slogan became: 'There is no such thing as a high risk group, just high risk behaviour'.

Around the same time in the late 1980s, the official nomenclature for the condition changed to 'HIV/AIDS'. 'HIV/AIDS' quickly became *de rigueur*, blotting out the distinction between cause and effect, and making infection itself the disease. By the late 1980s, the list of risk groups had become a list of risk behaviours. Behaviours that might lead the person to engage in 'risky' sex, such as excessive drinking or recreational drugs, even 'AIDS fatigue' or low self esteem, became 'causes' of HIV/AIDS. Thus risky behaviours – drinking, drug taking, 'excessive' sexual licence – were proscribed not as immoral but, in an apparently more rational, modern discourse, because they were bad for one's health (Alcabes, 2009).

However, the deconstruction of the notion of high-risk groups had disastrous consequences for gay men themselves. The message that 'everyone is at risk of AIDS', whilst true on a certain level, did not acknowledge that the level of that risk varied according to both (sexual) behaviour and the prevalence of HIV in the group from which one chose a sexual partner. The idea that everyone was *potentially* at risk from AIDS was mistakenly taken to mean that everyone was *equally* at risk. Even those gay men who had been involved in AIDS health education from the start of the epidemic colluded in this fantasy. They believed firstly that the only way to ensure adequate funding for services was to play down the fact that in the West it was very largely gay men who were contracting HIV. Secondly, they felt that the identification of homosexuality with illness and death encouraged a particularly poisonous form of homophobia.

HIV education and prevention efforts became mired in the language and mind-set of equal opportunities, whilst downplaying the fact that the epidemic had always disproportionately affected gay men in Britain, the USA and similar countries. This was dubbed the 'degaying of AIDS' (King, 1993). Whilst gay men continued to be sidelined in health promotion campaigns, and research was focussed on the danger of a future epidemic elsewhere, anger was growing in the gay community at what was seen as the mismanagement of HIV/AIDS funds, particularly for treatment and research. The radical AIDS activist movement was born in 1987, when Larry Kramer and others in New York formed the AIDS Coalition to Unleash Power (ACT UP), with its celebrated slogan SILENCE = DEATH.

One consequence of the 'de-gaying' of AIDS was that in countries like Britain and the USA, where gay men had always been the group at most significant risk of HIV, health promotion for gay men was wound down, with practically all the available resources going to groups at statistically negligible risk. For example, a survey carried out by the UK campaign group Gay Men Fighting AIDS in 1992 revealed that, of the 226 agencies with a remit for AIDS education in the UK, only 1.3 per cent had *ever* undertaken any kind of work for gay and bisexual men. Furthermore, when the envisaged AIDS epidemic did not occur in the heterosexual population, those funds that had been made available began to be cut (King, 1993).

In 1989, the AIDS education unit of the British Health Education Authority was closed down, as was the Cabinet subcommittee overseeing AIDS policy, and Mrs Thatcher personally vetoed a major academic study that was to have explored patterns of sexual behaviour. Both tabloid and broadsheet newspapers seized on the fact that AIDS was still a disease of gay men and not a threat to heterosexuals (Weeks, 1993).

From the early 1990s, a number of researchers around the world began producing reports of a so-called 'relapse' to unsafe sex amongst gay men (CDC, 2001). A number of factors appear to have been responsible for this. As health education began to be provided from the statutory sector rather than from the gay community itself, it began to seem less relevant to the target group and consequently less effective. The statutory agencies proved particularly squeamish about using language common to gay men themselves, and 'sex-positive' messages in campaigns were replaced with a more coy approach or with blatant scaremongering (King, 1993).

In the early 1990s, media representations continued to portray gay men as a threat, not only because they had (exclusively) promiscuous sex, went on sex holidays and had sex with bisexual husbands, but because they were selfish, wealthy and powerful, because they donated money to political action groups devoted to preventing mandatory testing, and were (metaphorically) 'in bed with' powerful political leaders (Booth, 2000). Occasional spikes of media interest in AIDS followed celebrity AIDS deaths such as that of singer Freddie Mercury in 1991, or the acknowledgement of the HIV-positive status of basketball player Earvin 'Magic' Johnson in the same year.

Until the middle of the 1990s, there was limited medical success in lowering the death rate from AIDS. However, in 1996, at the 12th International AIDS conference in Vancouver, Canada, euphoria greeted the presentation of results of trials of anti-retroviral treatment regimens containing new drugs – protease inhibitors – which, when taken in combination with the existing anti-HIV drug zidovudine (AZT) and other similar drugs, had the effect of reducing the AIDS death rate by

75 per cent (Gottlieb, 2001). These were originally dubbed 'combination therapy', a term later replaced with 'highly active anti-retroviral therapy' (HAART).

As a result of HAART, in the years following the Vancouver conference, specialist AIDS units and hospices across the Western world were closed as AIDS money was diverted from caring for the sick and dying to pay for new drug therapies to prevent those who were HIV positive from becoming ill. AIDS care in developed countries, which up to that point had been in practical terms often synonymous with palliative care, shifted its focus onto how to ensure adherence to difficult-to-take medication regimens.

As AIDS prognoses improved as a result of the new HAART, the distinction blurred between the categories of HIV positive, previously usually understood as HIV infected but well and not taking anti-HIV treatment, and AIDS, understood to mean ill with the complications of HIV-related immunosupression, taking anti-HIV and other treatments, and often approaching death. Those people with HIV/AIDS lucky enough to be able to access HAART had new challenges to face. They had to reconceptualise their lives, and to manage a practical and psychological transition from a self perception as suffering from a terminal illness to one of suffering from a chronic but manageable illness. For those with access to HAART, HIV/AIDS became a chronic disease, along the lines of diabetes, and new issues followed, such as maintaining the motivation to take life-long treatments while in good health, and practical issues such as returning to work.

By the end of the 1990s, HIV/AIDS was beginning to have the flavour of old news. The predicted heterosexual epidemic had not happened – the catastrophe in Africa did not count for the Western media as it could be explained away by 'cultural factors'. Anti-retroviral treatments now meant that in the West HIV/AIDS was not the death sentence it had seemed a decade earlier. Continuing high HIV prevalence in gay men confirmed the notion that AIDS would remain a disease of the *other*. Complacency about HIV prevention following medical breakthroughs in the treatment of AIDS meant that the syndrome was being reconceptualised as a chronic disease. The occasional media stories talked as much of 'AIDS survivors' as they did of 'AIDS victims' (Lupton, 1999a).

However, if the panic and hyperbole that characterised AIDS discourse in the middle of the 1980s was being replaced by complacency by the end of the 1990s, AIDS had still changed the scientific and cultural landscape. After AIDS, infectious diseases would be higher up the news agenda, and the topic of infectious diseases became linked with wider concerns about late modernity. The group of scientists and epidemiologists who coined the EID category in the late 1980s and early 1990s capitalised on this heightened interest in infectious diseases after AIDS to grab the attention of the media, the public and policy-makers.

The factors held responsible for the AIDS pandemic (sexual behaviour change, travel, commerce in wild animals, microbial adaptation of zoonoses due to deforestation, misuse of medical technology, nosocomial infections etc) were expanded into a wider list to include factors related to the 'emergence' of other infectious diseases, as explored in Chapter 1. These factors – human demographics and behaviour, technology and industry, economic development and land use, international travel and commerce, microbial adaptation and change, and the breakdown of public health measures – have been characterised as 'a list which was in many ways a wholesale condemnation of the consequences of modernity' (King, 2002: 768).

This notion that EID are a consequence of modernity is the polar opposite of the belief, widely held until the end of the 1970s, that modern biomedicine had conquered infectious diseases, and that they were a thing of the past. One strand of the discourse around EID therefore connects them with sociological theories around the consequences of modernity. The next chapter will therefore unpack the relationship between modernity and the emergence and re-emergence of infectious diseases.

4
Modernity, Globalisation and Emerging Infectious Diseases

As described in Chapter 2, the theory of epidemiological transition, first proposed by Omran in 1971, divides human history into epidemiological 'ages'. The theory argues that the first epidemiological transition occurred when hunter-gathering societies adopted agriculture about 10,000 years ago. This was followed by an extended 'age of pestilence and famine'. The next transition occurred from the end of the eighteenth century, in light of rising standards of living in more developed countries, where pandemics of infection began to recede and mortality rates began to fall. A similar transition was occurring in the twentieth century in developing countries. The theory proposed that, in the long term, across the world, pandemics of infection would progressively be displaced by degenerative and human-made diseases as the leading causes of death.

The epidemiological transition theory thus argued that different societies around the world were all inexorably progressing, albeit on different timescales, towards a future where infectious disease morbidity and mortality would be replaced by 'the diseases of civilisation', particularly heart disease and cancer. The emergence of AIDS and the re-emergence of other infectious diseases such as TB from the 1980s clearly pose a challenge to this theory. Some commentators have incorporated the emergence of new infectious diseases into the notion of epidemiological transitions and have argued that EID represent the latest epidemiological transition (see for example, Armelagos et al., 2005; Barrett et al., 1998; Weiss & McMichael, 2004).

Other writers have argued that the epidemiological transition model was simply wrong. Lewontin & Levins (2003), for example, argue that if proponents of the model had looked beyond the short time horizon of the past 150 years, they would have seen that every major change in society, in population, in land use, climate, nutrition or migration has prompted its own pattern of diseases. Secondly, if proponents of the epidemiological transition model had taken account of ecology, they would have seen that parasitism is a universal aspect of evolving life. Proponents of the epidemiological transition theory are charged with believing the myth of classical development theory: that 'development' would inevitably lead to worldwide prosperity and an increase in resources given to health.

The theory of epidemiological transition could thus be simply wrong, or the emergence and re-emergence of infectious diseases could be the latest epidemiological transition. Both views hold that just as earlier transitions were caused by changes in human society and technology, such as the adoption of agriculture, EID are caused by a range of factors related to modern human societies and contemporary technological advances. These factors – changes in human demographics and behaviour; technology and industry; economic development and land use; international travel and commerce; microbial adaptation and change and the breakdown of public health measures – bring us back to the original biomedical conception of the EID category as outlined in Chapter 1.

The concept of EID thus maps onto both theoretical conceptions of modernity *and* to the conceptual framework of epidemiological transitions (either by extending the theory or as proof that it was mistaken). Therefore this chapter will explore several different theoretical positions relating to modernity, particularly the increased theoretical attention given to risk, and relate those theories to EID.

Giddens and modernity

'Modernity' is usually taken to mean the era that started with the beginnings of industrial capitalism in Europe from about the eighteenth century, and refers to the type of political and social organisation that subsequently spread to the rest of the world. The modern era is characterised by a centred, hierarchical, Eurocentric, dominant worldview, and by a confidence in the inevitability of continuing human progress (Lemert, 1987).

Arguably the most influential theorist about modernity, contemporary social change and its impact on the self is the English sociologist Anthony Giddens. He argues that contemporary social changes are not a new era of *post*-modernity, but rather an acceleration of existing trends associated with modernity. He calls this *late* modernity, in which the consequences of modernity are becoming more radicalised and universalised than ever before. Thus, in his view, the Eurocentric worldview is losing its grip over the rest of the world not as a result of the diminution of Western institutions, but rather as a result of the logical extension of their global spread. This process is one of *globalisation:* 'the intensification of worldwide social relations which link distant localities in such a way that local happenings are shaped by events occurring many miles away and vice versa' (Giddens, 1990: 64).

In Giddens's reading, globalised late modern society is shaped by a number of factors. The first is a *separation of time and space,* so that 'far-flung' events can have an immediacy and impact over large distances. The point here is not that people are aware of events from other parts of the world of which they would previously have remained ignorant, but that the pooling of knowledge which is represented by 'the news' facilitates the global extension of the institutions of modernity.

In the context of 'far-flung' epidemic diseases, we can see that one of the institutions of late modernity – the global news media – makes people around the world aware of localised epidemics of infectious disease, such as the outbreak of bubonic plague in China in 2009, for example. This awareness facilitates another institution of modernity – international bodies such as the WHO – in strengthening global epidemiological surveillance, in effect over the heads of the governments of the nation states involved. This trumping of national sovereignty is justified on the grounds that it is the only way to prevent the spreading of epidemics via yet another aspect of our globalised and interconnected world – easy air travel.

The second factor shaping late modern societies relates to this notion of *time-space distanciation:* it is the idea that societies develop what Giddens calls *disembedding mechanisms,* by which social activities are 'lifted out' from their localised contexts and are reorganised across time and space.

An example this kind of disembedding mechanism in terms of emerging infectious diseases would be the way that contemporary globalised food production facilitates the spread of often difficult-to-trace food poisoning outbreaks. As described in Chapter 1, in earlier modern modes of food production, food was generally produced more locally and its consumption was generally limited to a certain time frame after its production. In late modern society, packaged food might contain ingredients from several continents, produced out of season, shipped across the world to be processed and then perhaps shipped on to other countries before it reaches consumers' plates. Furthermore, as well as food *production* being globalised, in late modern society food *culture* is also increasingly stripped of any localised context, so that it is entirely unremarkable to drink a Starbucks cappuccino (American? Italian?) in Moscow, to eat pizza in a 'back-packers' café anywhere in the developing world, or to eat a Thai or Indian curry in a 'traditional' English country pub.

Another social change associated with late modernity is the breaking down of traditional norms and values, with increasingly individualised lives and fragmented family structures, often stretched over continents and across the generations. Giddens is particularly interested in how these types of social changes impact on the self. An important theme in his conception of late modernity is the reflexive nature of modern social life. He contrasts how in traditional societies people might expect to blindly follow a role or identity marked out for them, whereas in late modern societies, individuals are surrounded by doubt and change, and have to engage in a reflexive construction of the self.

While people in pre-modern societies were guided by the 'expert' knowledge of, for example, religious leaders, they could potentially ignore that advice and still function in their daily lives. However, in late modern society, our relationship with 'expert' knowledge has changed to the extent that we cannot, in the same way, completely opt out of the abstract systems involved in our institutions. In modern society our 'experts' – doctors, scientists, economists, sociologists, psychologists and so on – are constantly re-examining our social practices. Our institutions and practices are then continually reformed and altered in the light of this incoming 'expert opinion' and new 'knowledge' about those very practices. This *reflexive appropriation of knowledge* – wherein the production of knowledge about social life becomes integral to the reproduction of that system – has the effect of sweeping away the fixities of *all* traditional types of social order (Giddens, 1990; Giddens, 1991).

Another central concept of late modernity is globalisation. Globalisation can mean many things. It can be taken to mean cultural globalisation, namely the flow of information, symbols, 'lifestyles' and so on around the world, which is usually characterised as 'Americanisation' or 'McDonaldization' (Smith, 2001). Multinational corporations and brands such as Nike, MTV, Disney, General Motors, Microsoft, Pepsi, Coke and so on are perhaps more accurately understood as transnational, post-national or even antinational, as they abandon the very idea of nation. These multinationals do not recognise foreign countries as *foreign*; for them and their consumers there is only one world and it is 'McWorld' (Barber, 1995).

Related to this soft cultural imperialism, globalisation can also be thought of in terms of politics, particularly the way that the borders of the nation state are being dissolved and superseded by organisations such as the United Nations and the European Union. However, for many commentators, globalisation is primarily an economic force, implying that (nearly) all national economies are now networked with other economies around the world through international financial markets, free trade zones and multinational corporations.

One feature of globalisation, contingent on its economic and political aspects, is the phenomenon of mass migration. Whilst there have always been population migrations, and merchants would have travelled long distances in pre-modern times, most people in pre-modern societies were relatively immobile and isolated. In contrast, late modernity is marked by the ease of modern travel and the enormous mobility of people. Transport barriers have been reduced, first by the nineteenth-century succession of steamships over sail, and then in the twentieth century by the growth of civil aviation. This has lead to a 1,000-fold increase in spatial mobility, for leisure (for the rich), or in the form of migration as a result of economic and social upheavals (for both rich and poor), with half of that rise coming since 1960. Simultaneously, over the past 200 years, the human population has grown sevenfold from less than a billion to over six billion, and half of that increase has been in the last 40 years (Cliff & Haggett, 2004).

This collapse of geographical space, combined with population growth, has had profound effects on the circulation of human populations and has allowed a greatly increased traffic of infectious diseases. For example, the average time between symptoms of measles appearing in one person and symptoms appearing in another person directly infected from the first – a measles 'generation' – is 14 days. Whereas in the early nineteenth century, the sea route between England and Australia took a year, by the early twentieth century steamships took less than 50 days, reducing the number of measles generations *en route* from six to three. By the mid to late twentieth century air travel had further reduced the travel time for the same journey to 24 hours, thus greatly increasing the chances of measles surviving on board and of infected people reaching Australia (Cliff & Haggett, 2004).

Another consequence of the mobility afforded by modern forms of transportation, combined with advances in technology such as television and the Internet, is that it gives both rich and poor an awareness of other, previously distant, ways of life. Giddens draws particular attention to the links between *reflexive modernity* and contemporary societies' changing relationship with risk, particularly the way that the circularity of the reflexive character of the self, the social institutions of modernity and the forces of globalisation all combine to form a universe of events in which risk and hazard take on a novel character (Giddens, 1990). Here both Giddens and the social theorist Ulrich Beck arrive independently at a similar theoretical position relating to the contemporary concern with risk and trust in scientific expertise.

Different models of risk

Risk is arguably one of the most important themes in contemporary social science, and different notions of risk diverge from many different theoretical starting points. Before exploring Giddens' and Beck's model of risk in late modernity, it is worth unpacking these different ways in which risk has been conceptualised in the different social sciences.

As discussed in Chapter 2, in the twentieth century, there was an enormous reduction in the *risk* that a person would die early (in a developed country at least) from an infectious disease. The word *risk* is used in this sense to mean the probability that something bad will happen to you – no one talks of 'the risk' that they might live to enjoy a healthy and disease-free old age. In this *realist model of risk,* risk is seen as an objective hazard, threat or danger. Although proponents of the view that the risks we face are *real* would acknowledge that risks may be distorted through social or cultural interpretation, they would still argue that risk can be measured and quantified independently of social or cultural forces (Lupton, 1999b).

The techno-scientific literature is steeped in this realist position. In medical journals, for example, the calculations that 'experts' provide about risk tend to be treated as if they were value-free, unbiased, objective facts. There is often a thinly disguised contempt for laypeople's 'difficulty in understanding' risks. An example here might be the way that, in biomedical literature, the public's concerns about the risk of the MMR vaccination were bemoaned as leading to unvaccinated children left at risk of the complications of measles. The implication in this realist conception of risk is that there is some sort of Platonic standard or risk scale that exists 'out there', based on science or statistics that can be used to judge how right or wrong a specific estimate of a risk is.

Much of the social scientific literature on risk perception inherits this starting point and sets out to 'test' perceptions of risk, for example through surveys and questionnaires. Risk perceptions are then seen as being 'faulty' or 'deficient' if they do not concur with an expert analysis of that risk. One criticism made of this *realist* risk perspective is that it seems to posit risk assessments as being made solely on an individual basis and underplays the role of influence from the wider culture. The problem with this *realist* perspective then is that it treats science and risk as though they were independent of sociocultural influences and effects (Lupton, 1999b). This concern is taken up in various ways by those who argue that risk is socially constructed.

One strand of social constructionism stands diametrically opposed to the *realist* model. The *strong constructionist model* of risk, deriving largely from the work of Foucault, argues that the discourses (the language and practices used) and the institutions around a phenomenon such as risk serve to bring the risk into being, to construct it as a phenomenon. From this perspective, nothing is a risk in itself. Rather, what we understand to be a 'risk' is a product of historically, socially and politically contingent 'ways of seeing'. This model thus focuses on how discourses construct notions of realities, meanings and understanding. For the *strong constructionists*, expert opinion provides the advice and guidelines by which people are compared against norms, trained and rendered productive. For Foucauldians, this discourse of risk – called *governmentality* – is thus a way of promoting the self-surveillance and self-regulation of people and populations. Through the efforts of statisticians, epidemiologists, lawyers and so on, people are identified as being 'at risk', and thus requiring particular forms of intervention (Lupton, 1999b).

Whilst this *strong constructionist model* of risk has been used in various ways by Foucauldians to critique medicine, social scientists generally tend to frame the media discourse around EID in terms of a weaker form of social constructionism. This *weak constructionist model* of risk (Lupton, 1999b) sees risks as existing as objective hazards, but argues they cannot be known in isolation from the social and cultural processes that inevitably mediate them. Unlike the *strong constructionist model*, this weaker form of social constructionism would not argue about the *realities* of the risks we may face. It would instead focus on what meanings are attributed to risks and how and by whom the risks we are said to face are selected for attention and politicised. One strand of this *weak constructionist model* is the *critical structuralist* work of Giddens and Beck. Another strand of *weak constructionism* in the risk literature is the *functional structuralist* approach of the English cultural anthropologist Mary Douglas.

To say that some phenomenon or other is a social construction often attracts the ire of people who take social constructionism to mean that what is being said is that the phenomenon is somehow less *real*, or that it is diminished or dissolved in some postmodern sense. To say HIV/AIDS is socially constructed, at least in the *weaker* sense, does *not* mean that people do not suffer and die from acquired immune deficiency syndrome. It *does* mean the discourse that grew up around AIDS, as a 'gay plague' for example, constructs our thoughts about the *reality* of the medical syndrome in certain ways. Furthermore, the underlying social tensions that inform the choice of language are exposed by analysing the discourses around infectious diseases. As discussed in the previous chapter, the social construction of AIDS, for example, was built on the concerns of the religious right about the liberalisation of attitudes to homosexuality in the 1970s. To think of AIDS, and indeed all EID, as social constructs in this way is particularly fruitful because it begs the question as to whose purposes and what *functions* these constructions serve.

The *Risk Society*

The German sociologist Ulrich Beck coined the term *Risk Society* to conceptualise contemporary society (Beck, 1986). Beck's notion of a *Risk Society* can be distinguished from that of others who might characterise contemporary society in terms of, say, a class society or an information society. Beck's central point is that, compared with the risks faced by people in pre-modern rural societies, or indeed in the early modern industrial societies, the *quality* of risks we face in contemporary societies is different.

Like Giddens, Beck argues that this is not a postmodern phenomenon. Rather than representing a radical break with modernity, the *Risk Society* marks the development of earlier modernity into a *more* modern world, sometimes called a 'second age of modernity'. 'It is not the crisis, but the *victory* of modernity, which through the logics of unintended and unknown side-effects undermines the basic institutions of first modernity' (Beck, 2006: 10).

For both Beck and Giddens, pre-modern concepts of risks, such as those posed by plagues and pestilence, derived from fatalism that saw the dangers as either God-given or as natural events. Later, in the early-modern industrialised societies of the nineteenth or early twentieth century, risks arose from factory-related or other occupational hazards, and were limited to certain localities or groups. Contemporary risks, such as global warming, derive from the reflexivity of modernity, insofar as they are produced by science and technology, and it is the scientists and 'experts' themselves who are called on to judge the safety of those risks.

According to Beck, these new types of *Risk Society* risks are characterised by three features. The first is that they are unbounded and de-localised, meaning that that their causes and consequences are not limited to one geographical location or space. This takes place spatially, insofar as new risks such as climate change do not respect borders; it takes place socially, in that because of the length of chains of effect, for example in financial crises such as the 'credit crunch', it becomes impossible to trace the causes and consequences of events; it also takes place temporally, in that contemporary risks have a long latency period. The second feature that characterises these new *kinds* of risk is their incalculability, so that their consequences are impossible to estimate scientifically. The final feature is that their consequences are deemed to be so catastrophic that the logic of making them more controllable through compensation breaks down. For example, the potential consequences of developments in human genetics are such that precaution is achieved only through prevention of the use of the technology (Beck, 2006).

Beck's roots are in the West German Green movement, so his *Risk Society* concerns are usually read as referring to environmental catastrophes, such as the nuclear accident at Chernobyl in the Ukraine in 1986. However, Beck's conception of *Risk Society* does *not* mean catastrophe. Risk, for Beck, means the *anticipation* of catastrophe. Indeed, once the anticipated risks become real, they cease to be risks and become catastrophes. Risk in the Beckian sense then moves elsewhere. For example, as discussed in Chapter 7, once a long-anticipated terrorist attack actually takes place, then new concerns come into focus: about the use of new tactics such as bioterrorism, the effect of the attack on markets and so on.

> Risks are always events that are threatening. Without techniques of visualisation, without symbolic forms, without mass media etc, risks are nothing at all. In other words, it is irrelevant whether we live in a world which is in fact or in some sense 'objectively' safer than all other worlds; if destruction and disasters are anticipated, then that produces a compulsion to act. (Beck, 2006: 4)

Although the examples Beck gives are generally environmental, the *Risk Society* model also fits the risks said to be posed by EID. As described above, the nature of contemporary food production means that food risks are no longer limited geographically, and, as will be discussed in the next chapter, the spread of epidemics such as SARS are facilitated by the ease of modern travel. Many EID, including AIDS and 'mad cow disease' are characterised by a long latency period, and the latter also gives an example of the incalculability of these contemporary threats from infectious diseases.

So for Beck, and perhaps to a lesser extent for Giddens, risk and uncertainty arise from the realisation that the certainties and hopes of the utopian project of modernity are not being realised. As discussed in subsequent chapters, in many ways the media coverage of the risk of EID, particularly after AIDS, seems to follow this *Risk Society* model, highlighting wider contemporary public anxieties, in particular anxieties *both* about the apparent inability of technology (and biomedicine) to contain new threats posed by infectious diseases *and* concerns about globalisation aiding their spread.

As discussed above, one of the consequences of economic globalisation is the unprecedented global movements of people. This population movement is largely a result of increasing inequalities between the sparsely populated and rich countries of the north and the densely populated and impoverished countries of the south. Multinational companies spread across national boundaries and continents and move to where the poor and unemployed live; those with sought-after job skills migrate to where they can make the most of them, and the poor move to where 'milk and honey beckon' (Beck, 2000). Beck is particularly interested in this feature of late modernity: the weakening of the nation state, which allows for greater mobility of workplaces and people.

Mary Douglas and risk

Giddens and Beck both argue that contemporary risks are thought to arise as a result of human action and the reflexivity of modernity. They both contrast contemporary conceptions of risk to risks in pre-modern times, which were greeted with fatalism as either God-given or natural events. Another strand of *weak constructionism*, deriving from the work of the English cultural anthropologist Mary Douglas, argues that the risks we face in modern societies, or at least the 'modern' reactions to those risks, are similar to those that can be found in what she calls 'primitive' societies. Douglas's earlier work *Purity and Danger* will be discussed at length in Chapter 6. Here, the discussion focuses on her later work on environment and risk, which has attracted renewed attention thanks to the increased interest in the *Risk Society*.

Douglas asks why some risks are highlighted more than others, unrelated to their 'objective' seriousness, quantified in terms of numbers of deaths associated with them. Her work is located within a Durkheimian tradition, which would argue that the cultural value of collective representations of real or impending disasters is that they *function* to maintain group solidarity, supplying groups of individuals with a common set of aims and objectives to protect themselves from a perceived danger. In addition, by identifying either outsiders, or less commonly privileged elites (*our leaders*), as the cause of the threat, people are provided with a shared outlet for their anxieties through casting the blame upon those who are identified as threatening to disrupt their way of life. Douglas focuses on how notions of risk are used to maintain conceptual boundaries between self and *other*. She emphasises how the concept of risk and the attribution of blame for a danger that threatens a particular social group is put to political use (Douglas & Wildavsky, 1982; Douglas, 1992).

While Giddens and Beck would highlight the uniqueness of late modern concerns about risk, for Douglas, the same blaming mechanisms are evident when 'moderns' are faced with a new threat as are evident in so-called 'primitive' societies. So, for example, when the new disease AIDS appeared, symbolic boundaries were constructed between healthy self and diseased *other* that functioned to apportion blame. The people in the category of *other* were then seen as responsible for the genesis of the disease; and/or for 'bringing it on themselves'; and/or for 'spreading' it. *Others* are dirty, have bizarre rituals and customs (injecting drugs, for example) and have perverted or promiscuous sex. As discussed in the following chapter, similar blaming mechanisms can be traced for other late-modern infectious diseases, such as 'mad cow disease' or SARS, which serve to confirm 'our' suspicions that *others* eat disgusting food.

For Douglas, the response to risk can thus be seen as a strategy for dealing with danger and *otherness*. Modern secular opinion would like to think that it sees nature as morally neutral and, by contrast, would see 'primitive' societies as dominated by superstition, with religious or supernatural explanations given to natural events, such as God's will or witchcraft. For example, plagues and other misfortunes such as floods, earthquakes and accidents are thought by 'primitive' peoples to be the result of sin or of the breaking of a taboo. Thus nature for 'primitive' societies is heavily politicised. Modern society, on the other hand, as exemplified by the *realist* model of risk, likes to think that it provides a rational, scientific, calculable explanation for misfortune.

Douglas argues that if this were indeed the case, 'moderns' would comprehend the risks they face as direct knowledge, as bare reality, and different from 'the clouded superstitions of the past'. Instead, she argues that just as in 'primitive' societies, in contemporary Western societies blame must be similarly attributed to every death, accident and misfortune. For her, the notion of risk in modern secular societies in explaining misfortune does the work of sin in pre-modern religious societies. Thus the modern, secular 'enlightened' view would argue, for example, that AIDS is not the result of sin but of 'risky behaviour'.

> On this subject we shall show that there is not much difference between modern times and ages past. They politicised nature by inventing mysterious connections between moral transgressions and natural disasters as well as by their selection among dangers. We moderns can do a lot of politicising merely by our selection of dangers. (Douglas & Wildavsky, 1982: 30)

Like Beck in his *Risk Society* thesis, Douglas sees the pre-eminence of risk at this point in history as connected to globalisation, as a consequence of which people feel that they are more interconnected and therefore more vulnerable to risks from *others* than they previously were. However, she cautions suspicion of environmentalists who focus on the perceived threat of an anticipated environmental catastrophe. For her, this apocalyptic scenario functions as a device for casting blame on *others*, who may be identified as a threat to 'us' or to our livelihoods (Wilkinson, 2001).

Although Beck and Douglas might disagree on the 'reality' of the risks we face, both conceive this reality as a social construction. Douglas's view of risk is thus similar to Beck's insofar as she agrees that there is a heightened and increasing risk awareness, and that the contemporary consciousness of risk is a consequence of late modernity and its attendant globalisation. However, for Beck our heightened awareness of risk is the result of a greater consciousness of risks produced by modern technology and its misuse, such as ecological risks. Douglas, on the other hand, is more of the view that our belief in, and our politicisation of, risk is due to greater social insecurity, in light of threats from *others* (David, 2005).

Douglas's notion of risk as a defence mechanism has its roots in psychoanalytic thinking, although she does not draw on psychoanalysis directly. Helene Joffe (1999) builds on Douglas's anthropological idea of in-group protection by linking the threat of danger with the *other*. Joffe arrives at a similar theoretical position, although as a psychologist, her interest is in how the identification with the group becomes embedded in the self. She is particularly interested in the ways in which laypeople make sense of the risk of infectious diseases and how their views are mediated by experts and journalists. According to her, the *Risk Society* does not necessarily leave people with a heightened state of anxiety. Rather, people have defence mechanisms, namely their representations of risks, that function to control anxiety.

For example, Joffe examined the consequences of AIDS-related blame for gay men, one of the out-groups constructed by the dominant group as *other* and she asks how this *othering* was experienced by gay men themselves. In interviews conducted in the early 1990s with British and South African gay men, she found that they shared the wider society's linking of their own identity to AIDS. As a consequence the gay men in her study viewed themselves negatively, highlighting how representations circulating in the cultural group via institutions such as the media can become internalised. This negativity was managed, in particular by the British gay men in her study, by externalising the blame for the origin and spread of AIDS in the form of conspiracy theories. These conspiracy theories not only located the blame for AIDS outside the gay community, but also created a sense of a shared enemy, rather in the way that the out-groups themselves are treated as the enemy of mainstream society (Joffe, 1999).

As noted in the previous chapter, the belief in conspiracy theories about the origin of AIDS was also prevalent amongst Africans, another marginalised group who were blamed for AIDS.

Othering and the new racism

The discussion of the *othering* in this context draws on Edward Said's (1978) account of *Orientalism*. Said argues that colonial hegemony was cemented by a series of binary oppositions that contrasted the rational West to an irrational, sexualised and childlike East. For him, the construction of identity involves establishing *others*, 'whose actuality is always subject to the continuous interpretation and re-interpretation of their differences from "us"' (Said, 1978: 332).

Orientalism is a collective notion identifying 'us' Europeans against 'those' non-Europeans, and advocating that European identity is superior to all the non-European peoples and cultures. The resulting portrait of 'us' and 'them' is reductive and 'invidiously ideological'; one in which the West is portrayed as

> rational, developed, humane, superior and the Orient, [...as...] aberrant, undeveloped, inferior... the Orient is at bottom something

either to be feared (the Yellow peril, the Mongol hordes, the brown dominions) or to be controlled (by pacification, research and development, [or] outright occupation wherever possible). (Said, 1978: 300–1)

Although Said's work focuses in particular on representations of the Orient, it fits into a wider debate encompassing Eurocentrism and racism. Eurocentrism (which encompasses the USA, Canada, Australia and so on) posits European life as central and non-European life as peripheral. Eurocentrism first emerged as a discursive rationale for colonialism and

bifurcates the world into 'the West and the rest' and organises our everyday language into binaristic hierarchies implicitly flattering to Europe: *our* 'nations,' *their* 'tribes'; *our* 'religions,'*their* 'superstitions'; *our* 'culture,' *their* 'folklore'; *our* 'art,' *their* 'artefacts'; *our* 'demonstrations,' *their* 'riots'; *our* 'defense,' *their* 'terrorism'. (Shohat & Stam, 1994: 2)

Modernism was characterised by the racist, hierarchical, Europeanised, dominant worldview against which was contrasted the difference of *others* (Lemert, 1987). Late modernity (or for some postmodernity) is, by contrast, marked by a shift away from biological ideas of racial superiority to a world view constructed instead on notions of cultural pluralism. Outright racism, posited on notions of the differences between 'racial' groups, has largely fallen out of fashion. It has been replaced by a view that different national or ethnic communities are neither superior nor inferior, better nor worse, dirtier nor cleaner, but *different*. Cultural difference is taken as a natural and unavoidable fact. This has been called the 'new racism' (Barker, 1981).

There are now approximately 120 million people who are living in countries other than those in which they were born. Particularly since the 1980s, migration has become synonymous with a new risk. Migrants have come to be regarded as a threat, rather than imperative to capitalist expansion. For example, in 1981 Canada welcomed 60,000 refugees, the so-called 'Vietnamese Boat People', but by 1999 there had been a dramatic shift in perception and the same country rejected 599 'Chinese Boat People'. Cultural differences are portrayed as threatening to 'our' way of life, and it is seen as rational to preserve one's culture through the exclusion of other groups. In this 'new racism', cultural pluralism is thought to lead inevitably to inter-ethnic conflict, which will dissolve the unity of the state. This modernises racism and makes it respectable, even amongst liberal academics and governments (Ibrahim, 2005).

In light of Douglas's view that notions of risk *function* to strengthen group solidarity, we can see that the ways that migrants and migration are resisted are often expressed in terms of the discourse that migration threatens the security of the host community. (This theme reoccurs more specifically in relation to EID, which are said to pose a threat to global security, as discussed in Chapter 8.) This new theorisation of race builds on 'genuine fears' of immigrants, not because they are bad, but because they are just different to 'us' and their presence threatens 'our way of life'.

This apparently innocent discourse does not even rely on dislike or blame of those different from 'us'. The new racism is theoretically bolstered by sociobiological notions that racism is a genetically pro-grammed evolutionary trait, a 'natural' extension of 'simple tribalism' or kin altruism. It argues that human nature is such that it is 'natural' to want to form a bounded community, aware of and separate from the cul-tural differences of others, and antagonism will be aroused if outsiders are admitted. Thus prejudice and xenophobia are cast as instinctual, innate and 'natural', and by linking race to nation/tradition the new racism is justified as neutral 'common-sense' (Barker, 1981).

As well as being expressed in terms of a threat to the culture ('the way of life') of the host community, on a more *realist* level, migrants are often said to pose a risk in terms of the infectious diseases they carry with them. Of course, concerns about immigrants bringing with them infectious diseases are nothing new. America saw its most intensive period of immigration between 1885 and 1910, leading to fears amongst native-born Americans that new immigrants were bringing with them or 'spreading' infectious diseases. For example, many doctors suggested that immigrants were bringing venereal disease into America and called for the restriction of immigration. Examinations at ports of entry failed to find a high incidence of venereal disease, but it was nevertheless sug-gested that most prostitutes in American cities were immigrants (Brandt, 1988). Italian immigrants were held to be the source of an outbreak of typhoid in Philadelphia in 1915 and of outbreaks of polio across east coast cities in 1916; Eastern European Jews became associated in the USA with TB, known as the 'Jewish disease' or the 'tailors disease'; As dis-cussed in the following chapter, the Chinese were blamed for outbreaks of smallpox and plague in West Coast cities.

In 1892, the US federal government opened a new immigration depot in New York harbor, Ellis Island. There, those immigrants found to be suffering from a so-called 'loathsome or contagious disease' that prevented them from supporting themselves, were denied entry to America (Kraut, 1994). By 1924, national origin was used as a means to justify exclusion of immigrants after Congress legislated to restrict immigration from certain southern and eastern European countries, based on their alleged genetic inferiority (Fairchild & Tynan, 1994).

The 1980s saw the greatest increase in legal migration to the USA since the 1920s and additionally as many as three million illegal immigrants were entering the USA every year. This fuelled fears of the burden they might place on the US health and welfare systems, particularly that immigrants with HIV and TB would cause a collapse in the Medicaid system (Fairchild, 2004). In an echo of the 1924 policy of excluding certain immigrants from 'dangerous nations', since 1987, the USA has prohibited entry to people with HIV, a policy which has been subject to widespread international criticism. This policy also had its roots in the fear that people from certain Caribbean and African nations may infect the US blood supply with HIV.

In 1991, the Bush administration simplified the visa waiver process for travellers, relying on individual travellers, mostly Europeans or Japanese who would be unlikely to become a burden on the US health system, to disclose whether they were HIV positive. People wanting to emigrate to the USA, the majority of whom between 1971 and 1990 came from the developing world, continued to be tested (Fairchild & Tynan, 1994).

Britain's colonial history has also led to similar fears of diseased immigrants. In the late nineteenth century, thousands of immigrants crowded into places like the East End of London, dubbed the 'bottleneck of Empire', which became home to almost 40 per cent of all refugees and immigrants in London. Almost all of the Jewish immigrants from Russia, who were poor, unskilled and ignorant of England, settled in the East End, where they could easily observe their religious laws, and find work, familiar habits, language and people. The terms 'immigrant' and 'Jew' became synonymous because of concerns about the social problems of the East End. By 1901, Russians and Poles (who were mostly Jewish but also included Catholics) comprised one-third of the total foreign population in the UK, although this was still only one-third of one per cent of the total population (Gainer, 1972).

The presence of these immigrants, and their association in the popular imagination with crime and disease, fuelled a Victorian anti-foreigner rhetoric, leading to the restriction of immigration to Britain through five Alien Acts introduced between 1905 and 1927 (Childers, 2005). These acts set the precedent for current UK immigration laws, and were meant to exclude undesirables: the diseased, the insane, the criminal, the putative public charge, and to accept the rest, including the genuine refugee from persecution. Although most of the Russians and Poles did pass inspection and entered Britain, the laws nevertheless had the effect of encouraging prospective immigrants to choose to go to the USA, where entry was more certain (Gainer, 1972).

After the demise of the British Empire, concerns about immigrants from the former colonies, and the diseases they were said to bring with them, gained renewed political momentum. From the late 1950s concerns were expressed that 'Asian' immigrants from the former colonies had high levels of TB. However, evidence suggests that rather than bringing TB with them, many immigrants may in fact have acquired the disease in poor and overcrowded housing in Britain after they arrived (Welshman, 2000).

The attitude to Commonwealth immigrants in the 1960s and 1970s resembled that towards Russian and Polish Jews at the end of the nineteenth century. In both cases, an ethnically homogenous society was undergoing rapid economic and social change and social mobility. The influx of immigrants was rapid and conspicuous, with economic competition exacerbating relations between immigrants and natives. In both cases the immigrant group was ambivalent about its attitude towards assimilation into British culture, being undecided whether to preserve its ethnic identity (Gainer, 1972).

Recent studies in North America, Western Europe and Australia attribute a large proportion of TB cases to the 'foreign born', who by 2000 accounted for 40 per cent of TB cases in the USA, about 50 per cent of cases in many European countries and 80 per cent in Australia. These figures have attracted the attention of anti-immigration groups in many countries. Studies of TB amongst recent immigrants to America found that it was transmitted in institutions such as refugee camps and holding facilities. Latent TB infections were also reactivated by the stresses faced during migration, such as poor overall health, poor nutrition and poor living conditions (King, 2003a).

However, media representations of TB in immigrant or established ethnic minority groups tend not to deal with such nuances. New Zealand's media, for example, focused on the TB threat posed by the migrant *other*, such as recent Vietnamese immigrants, with no or very little reporting of the links between socioeconomic determinants of health and TB, or the difficulties that immigrants faced in securing housing and employment (Lawrence et al., 2008).

Similarly, the British national media's coverage of an outbreak of TB in a school in the city of Leicester in 2001 featured the suggestion that the global mobility of Leicester's South Asian population connected the city with areas where TB was endemic. In an echo of earlier colonial anxieties, immigration was again blamed for the increased incidence of TB, thus positioning the outbreak in relation to broader debates about globalisation and immigration. Whereas the local health officials and local media emphasised that the origins of the outbreak were unknown and speculation was therefore unwise, the national media represented Leicester as a borderless, post-colonial city with imperial connections to South Asia. The national media regarded this connection as 'common sense', the only possible explanation for the outbreak (Bell et al., 2006).

The mass media and the selection of risks

The increased movement of people is one consequence of the trend of the collapsing of geographical time and space in late modernity. Another is the accelerated globalisation of the flow of information via the mass media, which for most people in developed societies is the main source of their information about risks in general and infectious diseases in particular. The mass media are the cipher through which expert opinion is filtered and then, in the terms used by Giddens and Beck, feeds into the reflexive construction of self. The globalisation of the mass media is attendant on technical innovations such as the Internet, and on 24-hour television news services such as CNN, BBC World and Al-jazeera. The appearance of these novel technical innovations coincided with the re-emergence of infectious diseases as a 'new' threat.

In the 1980s, the way that news was reported began to change dramatically. In 1980, Ted Turner launched Cable News Network (CNN), the first 24-hour news channel, which became one of many new channels available via the new cable and satellite technology. Around the same time, technology was beginning to change the way television news was gathered. Previously, news reports were recorded using conventional film, which would then have to be developed in a laboratory. As video recording technology became increasingly sophisticated, it enabled news reports to be shot directly onto video without the need to subsequently develop the film. Similarly, as broadcast technologies became more sophisticated, these video reports were able to be transmitted live on air, rather than the film having to be physically transported to the news station to be broadcast.

By the early 1980s, the impact of new technologies meant that televisual news in particular was more diverse and more immediate, and there was more of it in terms of airtime. Similar technological innovations in news-gathering in print news media – faxes, computer typesetting and so on – also revolutionised print media in the 1980s. From the 1990s the Internet began to be widely available (for 'early adopters') and quickly gathered pace in terms of numbers of users, speed and amount of information available. Thus the history of infectious diseases from this point onwards becomes, to a much greater extent than before, a history of the media framing of those diseases, by which the public(s) collectively came to make sense of them.

The increased news coverage of infectious diseases begs the question of what impact the news has on its audience. Does the heightened awareness of the risk of infectious diseases that the worldwide news media makes possible actually increase audience/public anxiety, as Beck and Douglas would suggest? Or does the constant and increasing pitch of risk discourse in the news make people 'switch off' and distance themselves from what they may see as unthinkable or distant dangers?

Both Beck and Douglas have been criticised by those who argue that neither has made much effort to validate their theories in light of the empirical evidence on risk perception. Critics argue that the appeal of theories advanced by both Beck and Douglas lies more in their polemical functions than in the extent to which they rely on empirically supported research on how the public acquire and interpret media perceptions of risks. Such research points to a considerably more complex picture:

> [D]espite the considerable analytical investment which Beck makes into the alleged role of the mass media in 'sounding the alarm' about the reality of hazards ... [s]o far Beck has made very little attempt to engage with the literature of communication research, and further, he appears to be largely unaware of the difficulty of theorizing the effects of mass media in light of the discovery of audience studies. (Wilkinson, 2001: 12)

As Douglas would have it, 'moderns' politicise nature by the selection of risks. Who then decides which diseases are newsworthy, and on what criteria are these decisions based? The best predictor of news coverage in developed countries is that a disease poses a risk to people of the same demographic profile as the imagined audience – read white, middle-class, heterosexual Westerners. Infectious diseases in 'far-flung' areas that affect only indigenous populations gain attention only when they affect wealthy people or foreigners. The closer to home the epidemic, the more likely the coverage. Once the agenda has been set, the media coverage Westernises the disease by referring to familiar metaphors – science fiction, crime, detective, mystery, apocalyptic or military metaphors (Moeller, 1999).

A similar point is made by Kitzinger & Reilly (1997), who examine which risks attract public attention and why the media pick up, and then drop, a particular risk issue. They conclude that the media are not simply reflecting a 'new epoch' (*à la* Beck) nor are they indiscriminately attracted to risk. Amongst the factors that influence the news media's attention to risks are: journalists' knowledge (some journalists shy away from stories where they have difficulty understanding the issues); news values and the need for 'real events' to serve as news hooks; the human interest factor (what they call the 'it could be you/it could be me' factor); the self-referential media momentum (by which once a story becomes newsworthy, other media outlets start to address it); and the amount of associated activity by pressure groups, professional bodies, politicians and so on.

Due in part to the success of the EID category, as well as to the growth of the new globalised news media, in the 1990s infectious diseases moved up the news agenda, as each new epidemic or threatened epidemic accumulated to create an increasing pitch to the discourse of risk that infectious diseases posed. As with AIDS, the social constructions of each new disease have their foundations both in the existing historical and metaphoric landscape, for example the use of the plague metaphor, as well as in underlying social tensions, such as unease about mass migration or liberalisation of attitudes concerning sex and sexuality.

Concerns about the direction of late modern society thus have their meanings transferred onto the new epidemics, until EID became a metaphor for modernity itself. Furthermore, these trends are cumulative, and therefore the following chapter will examine how these post-EID category risks of infectious diseases, including Ebola, 'mad cow disease', SARS, and 'superbugs', became increasingly politicised from the 1990s onwards.

5

Mad Cows, Modern Plagues and Superbugs

From the 1990s onwards, there was an exponential increase in the media coverage of emerging infectious diseases. In the USA, there were several media scares following localized outbreaks of infectious diseases previously seen very rarely, or not at all. For instance, in 1993, the largest-known cryptosporidiosis outbreak occurred at water treatment plants in Milwaukee, Wisconsin, with an estimated 403,000 people affected and 54 deaths (Hewitt & Schmid, 2002). In 1995, several Texan youths contracted Dengue fever after a camping trip in a Mexican border town (Holtzclaw, 2002). In 1996, an outbreak of food poisoning caused by Guatemalan raspberries contaminated with *Cyclospora cayetanesis* affected 1,465 people in the USA and Canada (Lashley, 2002). Most famously, in 1999, an outbreak of West Nile virus occurred in New York, the first identification of the disease in the Western hemisphere.

The discussion here, however, focuses on other diseases that gained particular significance and came to epitomise the new EID category. The first of these was so-called 'mad cow disease', which in 1996 was linked to disease in humans. At around the same time, a 'far-flung' epidemic of Ebola garnered a huge amount of media interest. Through the 1990s and early 2000s, the issue of 'superbugs' gained momentum in both political and media circles. The late 1990s also saw increasing attention focused on the risk of a potential global pandemic of highly pathogenic avian influenza (HPAI) from the H5N1 strain of influenza originating in South East Asia. However, it was SARS, rather than H5N1, that caused global panic in 2003. Reportage of these various new diseases aggregated these stories (as 'emerging' diseases), and this cumulative effect led to a 'ratcheting up' of the risk discourse around them, as well as an increasing tendency to scapegoat and blame.

'Mad cow disease'

The 'mad cow disease' story began in April 1985 when a cow on a farm in southeast England became aggressive and developed problems with co-ordination. Despite various attempts at treatment, the animal died – as did seven more cows with similar symptoms on the same farm over the following 18 months. By 1987, similar cases had been confirmed in four other English herds, and the British journal *The Veterinary Record* published the first report of what was by then called bovine spongiform encephalopathy (BSE).

In 1988, as the number of cases continued to rise, the British government established the Southwood Committee to examine the problem. The committee concluded that BSE had its origins in a similar disease in sheep – scrapie – and had been transmitted to cattle through the practice of feeding them 'ruminant-based protein' (processed meat and bone from sheep and cattle). The use of such feeds was banned in May 1988, a measure that at the time was taken to protect animal health. The committee also recommended that BSE-infected animals should be compulsorily slaughtered and their carcasses destroyed. Farmers were to be paid 50 per cent of the market value of the animal, on the basis that a diseased cow was worth less than a healthy one.

Only in February 1990 did the government increase the compensation to full market price. Immediately, reported cases leapt by 75 per cent, evidence that, prior to this time, farmers had been sending diseased cows to market and thus into the human food chain (Weir & Beetham, 1998). In 1989, measures were introduced to exclude the most highly infective cattle organs and tissues from cattle older than six months from the human food chain. In the same year, the European Union (EU) restricted exports of cattle from Britain, the first of a number of restrictions placed on the export of cattle and beef.

The BSE crisis emerged at the end of a decade in which the credibility of the British government was already severely dented following several other food policy scandals (Lang, 1998). One of these was a rise in cases of food poisoning caused by a new, more virulent form of salmonella in eggs, which led to the resignation of a junior minister, Edwina Currie, after she said on television that 'most of the egg production in this country, sadly, is now infected with salmonella'. An inquiry followed, one of the outcomes of which was introduction of a new Food Safety Act in 1990 (Pennington, 2003).

Before 1990, there were very few reports about BSE in the British newspapers, and those occasional stories were usually confined to the science pages of the quality press (Gregory & Miller, 1998). These rare reports usually framed the new disease either as on a par with the salmonella scare – unpleasant, but not life-threatening for most people – or in terms of scrapie, a disease present for many hundreds of years in British sheep and yet one that did not pose a risk to human health (Washer, 2006).

The British news coverage of the BSE story first spiked in March 1990, when a domestic Siamese cat in Bristol was confirmed to have died of a 'scrapie-like' spongiform encephalopathy. Up to that point, the British government's line had been that BSE in cows was a derivative of scrapie. Yet although animals such as goats were susceptible to scrapie, cats were not, hence the ability of BSE to jump species to a cat was regarded as a cause for concern. During the following months, evidence began to accumulate for the incidence of spongiform encephalopathies in increasing numbers of animals, particularly zoo animals fed on meat and bonemeal (Lacey, 1994).

The British government attempted to divert attention from the crisis by trying to discredit dissenting opinion as scaremongering, and by vilifying scientists who argued that in the light of the mounting evidence what would later become known as 'the precautionary principle' should be applied to British beef. The government also shifted the blame for the collapse of the beef industry onto Europe. One of the most memorable images of the BSE story was a photo opportunity in which Agriculture Minister, John Gummer, fed a burger to his four-year-old daughter, Cordelia, in an effort to reassure the public. Such reassurances failed to satisfy other European states, who promptly banned British beef.

The British press, following the line set by the government, soon moved the debate away from the potential threat to health, focusing instead on the European ban and the government campaign against it (Miller, 1999). From its peak in the middle of 1990, media coverage declined, partly because the EU decided to allow British beef from certified BSE-free herds to re-enter the European market. Through the early 1990s, the British government attempted to banish doubts as to the safety of eating British beef to a degree that was 'politically stupid' (Lang, 1998).

In January 1994, a documentary was screened on British television about 15-year-old Victoria Rimmer, who was dying of Creutzfeldt-Jakob disease (CJD) (she died in 1996 aged 18). By the end of 1995, a further 11 possible cases in people under 50 years of age had been referred to the British health authorities. Eight turned out to have a new variant of Creutzfeldt-Jakob disease (vCJD). Whereas sporadic CJD is normally quite variable in symptoms and in the pattern of damage to the brain, these new cases were strikingly similar to each other. The vCJD cases also showed damage to similar areas of the brain as was found in cows with BSE (Dealler, 1996). In 1994, 18-year-old Stephen Churchill became the first to die of vCJD, although the cause of his death was not confirmed until the following year (Weir & Beetham, 1998).

After ten years of refusing to admit to any risk to the health of the public, the weight of evidence of a link between eating BSE-infected beef and contracting vCJD became too great for the government to deny any longer. On 20 March 1996, the Minister of Health, Stephen Dorrell, announced to Parliament that there was a 'probable' link between BSE and recent cases of vCJD in young people. The announcement caused a public outcry and a political crisis for the British government.

In the aftermath of the incident, the media was initially saturated with human interest stories about people who had contracted 'mad cow disease'. The most terrifying diseases are often those perceived not just as lethal but as literally dehumanising. In nineteenth-century France, for example, actual cases of rabies were both rare and inevitably fatal (before Pasteur's discovery of its cause). However, the rabies phobia that gripped people during this period involved countless pseudo-cases of infection by animals newly turned 'bestial', and even of 'spontaneous' rabies. There was a myth that rabies infection transformed people into maddened animals, unleashing uncontrollable sexual and blasphemous impulses (Sontag, 1989). A similar fear of becoming like a maddened, rabid animal pervades the coverage of 'mad cow disease' in 1996. Descriptions of the physical and mental decline of the young people who succumbed to the disease, juxtaposed with images of uncoordinated and frightened cows, made a clear link between the mad cow animal and the *once human being* (Washer, 2006).

Yet as in 1990, as the British beef industry collapsed, soon the emphasis of the British government and media again shifted away from the threat to human health and onto the European reaction and its threat to the domestic economy. The Conservative government of Mrs Thatcher, already intensely antagonistic to the EU, was furious at the bans on British beef, which it saw as a mask for protectionism of European beef markets.

The British C/conservative nationalism about beef was also related to the notion of beef as a traditional emblem of Britishness and a significant staple of the British diet, as in, for example, the traditional family ritual of the Sunday joint of roast beef and Yorkshire pudding. Other cultural identifiers include the 'Beefeaters' who guard the Tower of London, and the French nickname for the British: *les rosbifs* (Hinchliffe, 2000). Thus the attack on British beef by the French and Germans, of all people, was viewed by many as a continuation of centuries of mutual hostility. BSE therefore provoked a further deterioration in relationships between the UK and other EU member states.

Although the British reaction to the EU ban could be seen as xenophobic anachronism, the reactions of the Europeans were little better. For (continental) Europeans, the BSE story only confirmed their worst stereotypes about terrible British food. As noted in the previous chapter, one way to distance the threat posed by a new epidemic is to blame *others* because 'they eat disgusting food'. Politicians in the EU addressed the problem of BSE as if it stood for *British* rather than *Bovine* Spongiform Encephalopathy (Brookes, 1999). Media coverage of the issue in the USA similarly depicted BSE as rooted in stuffy British identity and 'unnatural' norms. One ubiquitous pun used to distance the American reader from the BSE crisis was 'mad cows and Englishmen'. The British 'overindulgent' taste for beef was contrasted with 'not excessive' and 'healthy' American consumption of beef (Demko, 1998). From outside Britain, BSE was thus depicted as a problem for *others*, and not one that could happen 'over here'. (In 2003, BSE was found in cattle in Canada, and in the USA in a cow originating from Canada. The USA banned Canadian beef and cattle, and similar bans followed in Japan, South Korea and Taiwan (Broadway, 2008), causing major financial repercussions for Canada's farmers.)

If people outside Britain could blame BSE/vCJD on disgusting British food and 'excessive' British consumption of beef, what of the British themselves? The problem could not be distanced in the same way, as its origins were undeniably domestic. In Mary Douglas's terms, instead of the blame being directed *outwards* to *others,* the focus of blame for the British was directed *upwards* to privileged elites. The blame was placed unequivocally at the door of *our leaders* – the Conservative government – who for over ten years had reassured the British public that beef was safe to eat.

Another strand of this criticism related to the impropriety of the links between the Conservative Party and the farming and food lobbies. The National Farmers Union was an entrenched interest group in British government and policy-making; supposedly 'watchdog' bodies were dominated by members of Parliament with rural and farming interests (Weir & Beetham, 1998); there were several large-scale farmers in the Tory Cabinet and active in local Conservative constituency associations;

and many large food producers had also been generous donors to the Conservative Party (Grant, 1997).

As well as being directed upwards to *our leaders,* the blame for BSE/vCJD was also widely attributed to 'modern' farming methods, and in particular the practice of making carnivores of herbivores. In fact, the practice of feeding meat and bone meal to animals in Britain is not terribly 'modern' and dates back to at least the 1920s (The BSE Inquiry 2000). The term 'mad cow disease' was coined by David Brown, a journalist on the right-leaning broadsheet the *Daily Telegraph* (Gardner, 2008), although by May 1989 it had already begun to appear alongside 'BSE' in newspaper reports in both broadsheet and tabloid newspapers. The term clearly captured the *zeitgeist,* describing the 'mad' behaviour of the cows, as well as drawing on the metaphor of rabid 'mad dogs'. This image contrasts with the more customary images of cows, for example in children's stories or English pantomimes, where they are usually represented as placid and docile creatures.

In a certain sense, the 'madness' here refers not (only) to the diseased cattle, but also to a wider malaise of modernity (Leach, 1998). In Western societies, certain classes of animals – pets, primates and carnivores – are not considered food. The prohibition on eating carnivores may possibly stem from the fact that they potentially, albeit rarely, eat humans. The idea of incorporating an animal that may have itself incorporated human flesh is repugnant to Western sensibilities. From a Western perspective, 'primitive' peoples who eat what is considered 'non-food' – dogs, cats, monkeys – are marked as less 'civilised' and animalistic (Tiffin, 2007).

This horror also intersects with a contemporary discourse that condemns the mixing of genes from different species in genetically modified (GM) food. Eating cows that have been made carnivorous, and thus eating what is usually classified as non-food, is condemned as 'unnatural', as is the GM mixing of different categories. This echoes the food prohibitions of The Book of Leviticus (discussed in more detail in the following chapter), which classify certain things as unclean and not to be eaten, and condemns as unholy the confusion or mixing of different classes of foods (Scholten, 2007). There was thus a certain Biblical feel to the media descriptions of BSE as a punishment for 'unnatural' modern farming methods, for breaking a taboo by making 'cannibals' of cows.

As well as having echoes of the breaking of ancient taboos, 'mad cow disease' also seems a model *Risk Society* issue of late modernity. BSE was unbounded temporally in the Beckian sense, insofar as the prion proteins causing the disease persisted in the soil and resisted the normal sterilisation techniques used for surgical instruments. The risk was also unquantifiable, insofar as the consequences for human health from eating beef were very difficult to judge: epidemiological predictions of the scale of a vCJD epidemic at the time ranged from less than 100 to several million cases (Collinge, 1999).

Interestingly, although AIDS was an enormous media story in the UK when BSE was first reported around 1986, no links were made between the two diseases at the time. Only after the announcement of the BSE/vCJD link was made a decade later did the media frame for BSE change from salmonella to AIDS ('this could be *the next plague*', 'an epidemic on the scale of AIDS', etc). While the use of salmonella and scrapie to frame BSE in the early coverage acted to reassure and diminish the seriousness of the potential threat, the effect of the later framing of vCJD in terms of AIDS worked in precisely the opposite direction, amplifying the seriousness of the risk and the sense of fear (Washer, 2006).

BSE also seems a model *Risk Society* concern in that it necessitated dependency on expert judgement of the safety of beef, as BSE-infected meat did not look or smell any different from safe beef (Hinchliffe, 2000). Yet at the same time that very trust in expert opinion was damaged by the uncertainty and prevarication surrounding the communication of the risk.

Up to August 2009, there were 214 cases of confirmed vCJD, with 164 deaths, including three Britons who contracted the disease from blood transfusions. The majority of the cases were in Britain (165) and France (25), although cases were also diagnosed in other European countries, with three in the USA and one each in Canada, Japan and Saudi Arabia (The National Creutzfeldt-Jakob Disease Surveillance Unit, 2009). Media interest in 'mad cow disease' eventually waned, particularly in light of the growing newsworthiness of other EID.

Although the predicted epidemic of millions did not materialise, the story occasionally resurfaced in light of new scientific and epidemiological data, which indicated that the epidemic might already have spread, or had the potential to spread further. In 2004, for example, scientists announced that they had found the infectious agent of vCJD in a patient who had no signs of vCJD and who had died from an unrelated condition. He was thought to have been infected by a blood transfusion from a person who later developed vCJD. This suggested that as well as those previously known to have a susceptible genetic make-up, people with different gene types might also be vulnerable after a longer period of incubation (Peden et al., 2004).

Ebola

Around the same time that the link between BSE and vCJD was being announced, Ebola had resurfaced in Africa. As described in Chapter 1, 1976 saw the first reports of a 'new' disease, Ebola haemorrhagic fever, in the Sudan and Zaire. A second epidemic of Ebola in 1995–6 in Kikwit, Zaire, infected 316 people and caused 245 deaths. The first outbreak occurred before AIDS and the coining of the EID category; and before both Richard Preston and Laurie Garrett had brought the spectre of Ebola to public attention with their popular science books. While the first epidemic was largely ignored by the world's media, the second Ebola epidemic caused a media frenzy.

In his analysis of media coverage of EID, Ungar (1998) points out that the reporting usually follows a particular pattern, which he calls the *mutation-contagion* package. This is composed of the following core ideas:

- that *microbes are on the rampage* and that we are experiencing a 'wave of new assailants';
- that *microbes are cleverer than us* and, in a reversal of the idea that infectious diseases can be conquered, they are evolving to 'outwit us';
- that microbes and the environment are conjoined in an 'ecological parable' – arising from man-made issues such as population growth and antibiotic overuse;
- that *microbes know no boundaries* in a globalised world;
- and *that we are waiting for the next plague*.

This package is constructed around a frightening core of images and metaphors with little to reassure. However, the sense of threat is hypothetical, as the diseases remain abstract and affect geographically distant or marginal populations. At the same time, the reporting promises that 'medical progress' will contain and offset the threat, presenting a stream of 'amazing new discoveries'.

Ungar argues that the reporting of the 1996 Ebola epidemic in the Canadian, US and British media embodied many of the most terrifying aspects of this *mutation-contagion* package: a monster virus on a potential rampage, coming from 'elsewhere' and fitting the ecological parable. *All* of the media coverage paired Ebola with the words 'killer' or 'deadly', and almost all included descriptions of liquefying organs and profuse bleeding. While still distant for Western readers, Ebola was characterised as a harbinger of a possible wider pandemic. One feature of the Ebola reporting was the idea that the disease could be transported to Western countries in the bodies of those infected but without symptoms – the so-called *stepping off a plane scenario*. Yet very early on, the reporting changed to the *containment* package, 'erected on the metaphor of *otherness*', which diffused the potential panic. The exemplary protective methods of the Western experts were contrasted with the 'appalling sanitary conditions' of African hospitals. The focus of the threat was thus shifted from the virus itself to Africa's hospitals. After a few days, there was a further shift in the coverage, as attention was given to Western health teams – disease detectives – whose presence was contrasted with the chaos in Zaire. By this point Ebola was treated not as a rampaging virus, but rather as a disease that was difficult to catch. In particular, the *stepping off a plane scenario* was undermined, as journalists began to report that people with Ebola were not infectious until ill, and then unlikely to be travelling by plane (Ungar, 1998).

In the British newspapers, almost half of the coverage of the same Ebola outbreak linked the disease to monkeys or to the lack of appropriate African medical facilities. Beyond this, other factors implicated in the spread of Ebola were poverty, pollution, the forest environment and tribal rituals. By symbolising Ebola as essential to Africa as a whole, the coverage implied that such disasters were 'incontrovertibly African'. Africa was depicted as inevitably disaster-ridden, and the West, by implication, as superior. Ebola was compared with AIDS, with terrifying and horrific vivid descriptions of liquefying bodies. Readers were subsequently reassured with references to methods of containment of the virus by Western medical science. As with the coverage of African AIDS, the British media gave the impression of Africa as a 'cradle and hotbed' of disease, the 'dark continent' beset by famines, pestilence and primitive and perverse sexuality. Thus what the British readers already 'knew' about African AIDS led them to view Ebola in a detached way, by connecting it with the *other* (Joffe & Haarhoff, 2002).

As had been the case with AIDS in Africa, the Western news coverage of Ebola was pervaded by an emphasis on how the diseases could be brought under control only by Western science and Western doctors. At the same time coverage rarely gave Africans a voice, or alluded to the role they played. One rare study that does explore the views of people affected by Ebola examined how local residents viewed and responded to a later outbreak in 2000–2001 Ebola in Gulu, Uganda, one of the largest occurrences to date, with 425 presumed cases and 224 deaths (Hewlett & Amola, 2003).

The local Acholi people used three explanatory models to explain and respond to the Ebola 2001 outbreak. Initially, most families thought the symptoms of Ebola were the result of a bacterial infection or malaria and went to hospital seeking Western biomedical treatment, a model that had existed in the area for over a century. Symptoms were often treated with both biomedical and indigenous cures, for example with herbs from traditional healers, deriving from the indigenous concept of *jok* – spirits or gods from whom traditional healers, *ajwaka*, obtained their powers. As the symptoms continued, and the numbers of deaths began to grow, people realised that this outbreak was unusual and began to classify it using a third model – *gemo* – which in local folk belief was a mysterious bad spirit. Once an illness had been categorised as a *gemo*, a killer epidemic, the family were advised to quarantine the patient. The patient was moved to a marked house at least 100 metres from other houses, no visitors were allowed, everyone's movements were limited, and only survivors of the same illness were allowed to care for them. If the patient recovered, they had to wait a full lunar cycle before being allowed back into the village. If they died they were buried at the edge of the village (Hewlett & Amola, 2003).

Despite their similarity to Western biomedical notions of epidemic control, Acholi elders were adamant that these practices preceded contact with Westerners in the late 1800s. Thus indigenous epidemic control measures were consistent with those being promoted by Western healthcare workers. Although some cultural practices, such as those surrounding burial, did amplify the Ebola outbreak, most people were willing to modify these and co-operate with Western healthcare workers. WHO staff were concerned that local people with symptoms of Ebola were not coming to the hospital, and believed that it was because they were afraid of being buried there and not in their village if they died. However, locals ran from the ambulances not because they were afraid of being buried outside the village, which would have happened in their indigenous system, but because they were suspicious of white people, whom they commonly believed were buying and selling and body parts (Hewlett & Amola, 2003).

'Superbugs'

By the middle of the 1990s the emergence of 'superbugs' was also beginning to gain increasing media attention. Occasional flurries of media reporting thus followed stories such as 'flesh-eating bacteria' (Gwyn, 1999) or the diarrhoea-causing 'new superbug' *Clostridium difficile*

(Duerden, 2007). However, it was MRSA in particular that would become almost synonymous with the moniker 'superbug'.

Countries such as Scandinavia and Holland have remained relatively free of MRSA because of prudent antibiotic prescribing restrictions. Similarly, in some developing countries, such as The Gambia, there are low rates of resistance to due to reduced access to antibiotics. However, in others, such as Senegal, Nigeria and Vietnam, the unrestricted sale and use of antibiotics has led to antibiotic-resistant strains of bacteria (Farrar & Adegbola, 2005). Many hospitals in the tropics are like those in the 'pre-penicillin era', yet have a high prevalence of the antibiotic resistant bacteria of the twenty-first century (Shears, 2007). In the USA, the appearance of community-acquired MRSA (cMRSA) has caused widespread concern. cMRSA is transmitted not in healthcare settings, but for example, via sports activities and children's daycare centres. In the USA, MRSA infections rose to a new high in 2005, up nearly 30 per cent in one year, with 369,000 cases reported, of which about 5 per cent resulted in death (Spurgeon, 2007).

However, it was in Britain, which has one of the highest MRSA infection rates in Europe, that the issue became intensely politicised in Britain from the late 1990s, and particularly in the lead-up to the 2005 General Election, during which politicians used the issue to argue that only their party would adequately fund and manage the British National Health Service (NHS).

Political attention in Britain was focused not on what caused MRSA to evolve, such as the overprescription of antibiotics, but on why it was spreading, particularly as a result of allegedly poor hygiene in hospitals (Department of Health, 2004; Jones, 2004). The media largely reflected this bias, suggesting that by improving hospital hygiene MRSA could be controlled. In fact, although staphylococci can be found on hospital floors and other surfaces, they do not grow there and will gradually die. Cleaning or disinfecting a floor has only a short-lived effect as recontamination will soon occur, often in about an hour. The main route by which hospital infections are spread is on the hands of staff (Ayliffe & English, 2003).

Although the British media did not connect MRSA in any concrete way to the overprescription of antibiotics (by doctors) the media blamed MRSA on 'our' squandering of the medical breakthrough of antibiotics. This fits with Beck's *Risk Society* thesis, insofar as one of the features of risks in late modernity is that they are said to be caused by the misuse of technology, in this case antibiotics. The 'golden age of medicine' narrative describes antibiotics as one of the most tangible benefits of modern biomedical progress. In some respects, the MRSA coverage also fits with Ungar's (1998) model description of a *mutation-contagion* package above. However, in Ungar's model, the frightening 'bugs are evolving to outwit us' theme is offset with a promise of containment of the threat by way of 'medical progress'. In the media coverage of MRSA, there was no such promise of a medical solution for the problem, such as new antibiotics. The loss of faith in scientific medicine was evidenced by the numerous unconventional remedies reported in the media, of prophylactics that were said to protect against MRSA, or of homespun methods of 'boosting the immune system' (Washer & Joffe, 2006).

The metaphor 'superbug', like 'mad cow disease', makes concrete an abstract and invisible threat. Although the genesis of the term is unclear, it was used in the tabloids and broadsheet newspapers as early as 1985, originally in the context of stories about pesticides and the agricultural use of antibiotics. A widely publicised popular science book published in 1995 was called *Superbug: Nature's Revenge. Why Antibiotics Can Breed Disease* (Cannon, 1995). From about 1997 the term gained general currency and increasingly became synonymous with MRSA. Like 'mad cow disease', 'superbug' entered the lexicon and became widely used, even in political statements.

This begs the question: why 'super'? The origin of the word is from the Latin *supra*, meaning 'above' or 'beyond'. In idiomatic English, when combined with another word, 'super' means: 'to a great or extreme degree; extra large or of a higher kind, as in superstructure or super-abundant'. Whereas in American English 'bug' can refer to insects, in British English 'bug' only usually refers to germs. Thus 'superbug' combines 'super' with 'bug' and implies singularity, as in *supermodel*; strength, as in *superpower*; and/or indestructibility, as in *superhero*. In the 'superbug' discourse, there are ordinary 'bugs', for example the 'good bacteria' that colonise our gut and keep us healthy (as discussed in the following chapter), and then there are *superbugs*. MRSA is thus understood as a phenomenon that is ubiquitous, invisible, threatening and unconquerable.

If 'superbug' expressed the power of MRSA, then the calls by politicians and the media to 'bring back matron' implied nostalgia for a time when antibiotics were effective in containing disease and hospitals were clean and safe. 'Matron' is an anachronistic and explicitly gendered term, carrying with it connotations of matriarch, matronly and so on. For a British reader, the term would also carry a whole series of connotations related to the *Carry On* comedy films of the 1960s. The regimented female authority figure of the matron seemed a safer bet to sort out the MRSA crisis than the more neutral 'infection control nurse'. The matron figure symbolised a safe and trustworthy pair of hands for the NHS, with its associations of old-fashioned womanly hygiene, order and morality.

In the coverage of 'far-flung' diseases such as Ebola, and, as described below, SARS, there were graphic descriptions of the effects of the disease, but these tended to be impersonal ones: of liquefying bodies, lungs filling with fluid and so on. In the MRSA coverage, by contrast, there were many personal accounts of people's suffering as a result of the infection, including some of 'celebrity victims' who later become quasi-religious in their crusades against MRSA (Strong, 1990). The human interest factor in MRSA was constructed around an assumption that 'it could be you or me'. This human interest factor was not an intrinsic quality of the risk of MRSA, or of the 'flesh-eating bug' story, but was a construct related to journalists' perceptions of their audiences and their own identities (Kitzinger & Reilly, 1997). In other words, the journalists assumed that the plight of the human face given to MRSA would reflect and resonate with the audience and thus generate empathy.

This politicisation of MRSA recalls Mary Douglas' observation of how modern societies politicise risks by selection, whereas 'primitive' societies invent causal connections between natural events and moral transgressions, in order to cast blame. Like 'mad cow disease', 'superbugs' could not be represented as geographically distant from a British perspective, and unlike AIDS or Ebola superbugs did not only affect *others*. Thus the blaming/*othering* model seen in the distancing responses to other infectious diseases could not be applied in the case of MRSA. Instead, as with the 'mad cow disease', when the blame could not be directed outwards at *others* it was directed upwards to *our leaders* and thus became an issue in the 2005 election.

'Hong Kong' flu

The late 1990s also saw increasing global attention being turned toward South East Asia, and to what was considered an inevitable pandemic caused by a new strain of influenza which was expected to emerge from there.

All the influenza pandemics that have been traced to their source (since 1888) have been found to have their origins in China's Southern Guangdong (Canton) Province. This is attributed to the system of farming there, devised in the seventeenth century, in which rice farmers use ducks to keep flooded rice fields free of weeds and insects. As the rice blossoms, the ducks are put on waterways and ponds, and, after harvesting, they are put back on the fields, where they eat the remaining grains of rice, and are thus fattened for the table (Kolata, 1999). The farmers also keep pigs alongside the ducks, and since pigs can be infected with both avian and human influenza strains, genetic material from avian strains of influenza is sometimes transferred to strains that are infectious to humans via swine by a process known as reassortment or antigenic shift.

The potential of avian influenza to infect humans is exacerbated by the practice of importing chickens into Hong Kong from mainland China, where they are kept alive in food markets and only slaughtered on the request of the customer when buying the chicken. This traditional ritual is maintained because the Chinese value the freshness of food (Joffe & Lee, 2004).

Influenza viruses continually circulate in humans and cause yearly winter epidemics, but novel strains emerge sporadically every ten to 40 years as influenza pandemics that can infect between 20 to 40 per cent of the world's population in a single year (Taubenberger et al., 2001). As noted in Chapter 2, the worst pandemic in recorded history, with a greater death toll than even the Black Death, was that of the 1918 'Spanish flu'. Further pandemics derived from avian influenza strains followed in 1957, when H2N2, or 'Asian flu', travelled east along the routes of the Trans-Siberian Railway from China and Hong Kong into the Soviet Union, and west by sea from Hong Kong to Singapore and Japan and soon after to the USA, where it remained prevalent for ten years. In 1968, a less severe pandemic of H3N2, 'Hong Kong flu', travelled a similar route to the 1957 pandemic, spreading outwards from Southeast Asia (Kitler et al., 2002).

Until 1997, there was no evidence that a wholly avian influenza virus could infect humans directly. However, in May of that year in Hong Kong, a previously healthy three-year-old boy died from H5N1 'bird flu'. The avian strain, which had not been genetically reassorted in swine, infected 18 people in the territory, killing six. Although the virus was not transmitted between people, in December the Hong Kong authorities decided to cull approximately 1.6 million live fowl within the city environs and to ban the import of live birds from Guangdong Province. In 2001, the virus was again found in poultry in Hong Kong, prompting another cull of about 1.3 million fowl and a further ban on imports (Cyranoski, 2001).

In the years that followed, sporadic cases of H5N1 occurred in South East Asia, affecting birds and infecting humans, and there were more human deaths in 2004 and 2005 in Thailand and Vietnam, prompting further culls of millions of poultry. However, the first probable human-to-human case of H5N1 transmission occurred in September 2004 in a Thai mother who had nursed her dying child. By 2005, although only just under 100 people had died of H5N1, avian influenza was an almost daily feature of the US news (Davis, 2005). For example, in 1997, the year of the Hong Kong bird cull, there were 165 articles on the subject published in US newspapers and wire services, yet by 2005, the number of articles published had grown to 8698 (Trust for America's Health, 2006).

By August 2009, there had been 440 cases reported of H5N1 in people around the world, of which 262 people had died, with Indonesia and Vietnam being the worst affected countries (World Health Organization, 2009).

SARS

Yet while the global medical surveillance apparatus, and the global news media, watched South China in anticipation of a H5N1 'bird flu' pandemic starting there, another, unexpected, epidemic originated in the same region. At the end of 2002, cases of a new 'atypical pneumonia' began to be seen in rural China: the first appearance of the disease that was to become known as Severe Acute Respiratory Syndrome (SARS). SARS first came to the attention of the WHO at the end of February 2003 in Hanoi, Vietnam. Earlier that month, a doctor from Guangdong province in China had travelled to Hong Kong for a wedding and had unwittingly infected other residents at the Metropole Hotel. They carried the disease to Vietnam, and also to Singapore, Germany, Ireland and Canada. By the third week in March, several hundred people were infected, with cases reported in Hong Kong, Singapore, Toronto, New Jersey, California and Bangkok.

SARS is now known to be caused by a corona virus (SARS-CoV) and affected mostly adults, and only rarely children. Between two and seven days after infection, most people developed a high fever lasting three to seven days, with some patients developing other symptoms, including headache and body aches, or more rarely diarrhoea or mild respiratory symptoms. This initial mild period of the illness was followed by a period of breathlessness and chest pain. Most patients subsequently developed pneumonia, and around 15 per cent of those affected required artificial ventilation. There was a relatively high death rate of around five per cent. Transmission in healthcare settings was extremely high, and even in the first Hanoi cluster, infection rates of 50 per cent were reported amongst healthcare workers who had cared for SARS patients (Zambon & Nicholson, 2003).

The appearance of SARS provoked an immediate response from the global media. One of the most striking aspects of the SARS phenomenon was the speed at which the whole episode unfolded, from first reporting, to a screaming panic, to a rather embarrassed silence – all in just three months. Early reporting described the new threat as a 'killer' or 'deadly', and speculated as to how the epidemic would play itself out. The predictions were dire: 'this could be the next plague', the 'big one we've been waiting for' and so on (Washer, 2004). An important contextualising story for the SARS epidemic was the announcement, on 20 March 2003, that the second Gulf war had begun. Although there was some speculation at the outset that SARS may have been connected to bioterrorism, this was soon discounted. The epidemic therefore occurred around the same time as the US and British forces were invading Iraq, and the war may even have kept SARS out of the media to a certain extent.

The Western media reporting of SARS focussed on its effect on daily life, particularly in Hong Kong, the putative centre of the epidemic. The stories evoked either zombie or post-apocalypse horror-film imagery: deserted shopping malls, cinemas and restaurants; empty public transport; events where crowds would gather cancelled; and the use of surgical face masks. Initially, the Hong Kong authorities downplayed the danger of the disease, insisting that cases of 'atypical pneumonia' were confined to healthcare workers who had contracted the disease from an index patient (Baehr, 2006).

With the epidemic spreading, on 2 April, the WHO issued a travel advisory against non-essential visits to Hong Kong and to the Chinese province of Guangdong. As a result, Hong Kong became an 'international pariah' until the WHO removed it from its list of SARS affected areas on 23 June. Tourism plummeted and hotel occupancy in the territory fell by 20 per cent in April and May. Cathay Pacific, Hong Kong's flagship airline, which usually carried 33,000 passengers a day, was by April reduced to only 4000 passengers. Workers were laid off as over 3,800 businesses folded between March and the beginning of June (Baehr, 2006). Travel to other affected areas in East Asia was also reduced. In May, the decline in the numbers of passengers flying from London, Heathrow to Beijing was down 89 per cent, and to Hong Kong and Shanghai about 63 per cent (although the number of those going to Toronto declined only 20 per cent) (Lewison, 2008).

Apart from East Asian countries, the other place where SARS caused major problems was in Canada, particularly the city of Toronto, where there were 224 cases and 44 deaths, and nearly 30,000 people were quarantined by the Canadian public health authorities. The panic that accompanied SARS was unlike anything Canadians had ever experienced. Toronto's economy was numbed by fear, coupled with stigma and international travel sanctions (Feldberg, 2006). The origins of SARS in China led to boycotts of Chinese-Canadian businesses and prompted calls for the introduction of more stringent immigration controls (MacDougall, 2006). The outbreak of the disease in Toronto also exposed Canada's public health system, prompting the Canadian government to later review the nation's public health policy and infrastructure.

Later research indicates that SARS did not have the global economic impact that was feared at the time. In fact, the economies of Hong Kong, China and Vietnam all experienced faster overall annual growth patterns in 2003 than 2002. Although it is impossible to disentangle the impact of the fear of SARS from the fear of terrorism on the decline in travel to and from Canada, most of the decline in US international travel in the spring of 2003 reflected a fear of terrorism rather than SARS. Nor did the epidemic have other impacts in either South Asia or Canada – the trade in goods, supply chains and retail sales were all unaffected, as for every negative effect there was a potential offsetting response that mitigated the economic consequences (James & Sargent, 2006).

While the Chinese media talked of a 'war' on SARS, (Chiang & Duann, 2007) in the British press there was a striking lack of conventional military metaphors. This was probably attributable to the war in Iraq, which may have pushed commentators to develop a distinctive discursive system for the two stories (Larson et al., 2005; Wallis & Nerlich, 2005). Arguably, the Chinese media saw SARS as a threat to the Chinese nation in a way that it was not perceived to be elsewhere.

However, the general sense of pessimism emanating from the ongoing so-called 'war on terror' pervaded the Western reporting of SARS. There was a sense of an impending apocalypse, which was greeted with something approaching warmth, as if 'we' deserved it for 'interfering with nature'. The media compared the potential death toll of the SARS epidemic with the Black Death, the 'Spanish' flu of 1918 and the AIDS epidemic. This framing of the story in terms of epidemics with high death tolls, rather than say with the 'mad cow disease' or West Nile virus epidemics, which had much lower mortality, served to increase the sense of risk. Because of the tone of the news coverage, people who were far distant from the risk of SARS became concerned and started taking precautions as if they were in the affected area. Opinion surveys suggest that SARS had a significant psychological impact even in areas little affected, such as the USA, where there were only 75 cases and no deaths (Blendon et al., 2004).

According to the WHO, SARS was the first 'severe infectious disease to emerge in the globalised society of the twenty-first century' (World Health Organization, 2003c). This conceptualisation of SARS as linked to globalisation connects to Beck's *Risk Society* thesis. One of the characteristics of Beckian risks is that they are unbounded by the geography of the nation state. The concern was that SARS could be easily spread around the world through international air travel by infected passengers either transmitting the virus to those around them on the plane or taking the pathogen with them to another country: the *stepping off a plane scenario*.

In fact, although SARS was spread from one country to another by air travel, there is evidence that in-flight transmission to other passengers was uncommon. For example, German researchers traced 39 passengers who had travelled within four rows of a man who had flown from Hong Kong to Frankfurt on 30 March and who later developed SARS. All the 39 passengers' blood samples tested negative for SARS antibodies (Breugelmans et al., 2004).

If from a Beckian perspective SARS can be cast as a phenomenon of the late modern globalised era, then from Douglas' perspective, the reactions to SARS resonate with epidemics that struck 'primitive' societies, particularly the way that *others* were blamed and scapegoated. International media coverage of SARS (excluding that of China its supporters), consistently blamed SARS on the mainland Chinese people and the Chinese Communist system.

This blame was directed on several fronts. Firstly, the Chinese Communist authorities were blamed for having covered up the scale of the epidemic and for not having 'co-operated' with the 'global health authorities', namely the Western doctors, scientists and epidemiologists of the WHO. The Chinese were stereotyped as corrupt and mendacious in the Western media, and Chinese 'secrecy' was in turn linked to the purported 'personality' of the Chinese system and its 'habit' of avoiding or denying sensitive or negative issues, with the analogy given of China's mismanagement of its HIV epidemic (Buus & Olsson, 2006; Chiang & Duann, 2007; Washer, 2004).

A second strand of blame related to certain (Chinese) individuals. The doctor at the centre of the outbreak at the Hotel Metropole, Dr Liu Jianlun, was described in the media as *patient zero*. The origins of the term are in the AIDS epidemic, in which, as described in Chapter 3, a Canadian air steward was said to have recklessly transmitted HIV to many of the early North American cases. The term *patient zero* seems to have entered the lexicon, as it was used in the media accounts of SARS without any further explanation. Dr Jianlun was, with others, also described as a *super-spreader*, and, together with some other individuals, was blamed for carelessly 'spreading' the disease, for example by travelling to Hong Kong after caring for SARS patients in China.

However, the most prominent element of blame was directed against the Chinese people and Chinese culture more generally. The Chinese were said to be fond of exotic foods, to live close to animals, and to have poor hygiene practices. Singled out for criticism were the alleged Chinese habit of spitting in public places and China's unhygienic live animal markets. Even in the more liberal British broadsheets, there was a coherent package of themes relating to dirt and difference, clearly meant to invoke 'our' disgust at the way 'they' live and what 'they' eat. The British reader, assumed to be not of Chinese origin, was thus led to place the responsibility for SARS at the door of the Chinese. The recurring theme of *'others* are dirty / eat disgusting food' again had the effect of reassuring that 'it couldn't happen here' because 'we' don't live like that (Washer, 2004).

In the Western media coverage, reflecting the treatment of Africans in the coverage of AIDS and Ebola, the Chinese themselves were rendered invisible, seldom quoted, and their opinions rarely sought. For example, while the WHO press release reporting the death of Dr Carlo Urbani stated that he was the 'first WHO officer to identify the outbreak of this new disease' (World Health Organization, 2003b), in the newspaper reports he was credited with being 'the first person' to identify the disease. The newspapers actually meant the first *Westerner* rather than the first person. Yet when the newspapers accused the Chinese of a cover-up, they were implicitly acknowledging that Chinese doctors must have identified SARS as a new disease several weeks or months earlier.

A whole set of images and symbols were used repeatedly in the Western reporting of SARS that spoke of Chinese irrationality, backwardness and chaos, and of the threat this posed to the rationality and superiority of the West. China, the Chinese and their culture thus threatened 'global' (read Western) health and institutions. The possibility of containment was provided by another set of images: heroic Western doctors, laboratories and surveillance, with their associated connotations of rationality, modernity and order.

The binary oppositions of Western/Chinese images presented in the media coverage of SARS recall Shohat and Stam's (1994) point about *Eurocentrism*, discussed in the previous chapter. *Our* rational science was contrasted to *their* superstition; *our* global commerce (banks/airlines/shopping malls/multinational corporations) threatened by *their* chaotic, primitive and dirty markets; *our* surveillance thwarted by *their* secrecy; *our* efficiency (laboratories/doctors/scientists) battling *their* corruption. Poor Chinese peasants and the pathogens that they bred thus threatened to invade and lay ruin to *our* modernity (Washer, 2004).

In comparison to the lurid coverage of SARS in the Western press, the Communist Chinese mainland *The People's Daily* and Taiwanese *The United Daily News* (which supports a softer policy towards mainland China) used comparatively trivialising language, such as 'atypical pneumonia' to downplay the danger of the disease. *The People's Daily* constructed the disease SARS itself as the *other.* In contrast, the Taiwanese *The Liberty Times* (which supports independence for Taiwan) described SARS using the term *sha,* an innovated Taiwanese term triggered by the appearance of the similarly pronounced English acronym 'SARS'. This linked SARS to the commonly held Chinese folk belief that there are fierce gods, devils, ghosts or evil spirits – *shas* – everywhere. The *Liberty Times* depicted mainland China, and the people who travelled and did business there, as a menace, the source of *sha,* a combination of demon and invader attacking Taiwan (Chiang & Duann, 2007).

The blaming of the Chinese for the SARS epidemic builds on a nineteenth-century racist discourse which blamed the Chinese *other* for several disease epidemics. In the eyes of most nineteenth-century American whites, Chinese workers were regarded as little better than black slaves, heathen, primitive and morally degenerate. The Naturalization Act of 1870 limited American citizenship to 'white persons and persons of African descent', making the Chinese ineligible for citizenship, a status not changed until 1943 (Kraut, 1994).

The Chinese were blamed for the successive smallpox epidemics that struck San Francisco in 1868, 1876, 1881 and 1887 (Craddock, 1995; Craddock, 1998), and for the 1900 epidemic of bubonic plague in that city which killed 112 (mostly Chinese) people. During the 1870s and 1880s, there were concerns in the USA about the socioeconomic effects of the Chinese spreading diseases such as smallpox and plague, as well as of the spread of opium smoking and its relationship to prostitution and sexual behaviour (Ahmad, 2000). In 1882, the US Congress passed the Chinese Exclusion Act, which prevented Chinese immigration. Conventional (white) American wisdom of the day was that Asia and its living conditions were conducive to plague, as well as to other illnesses such as cholera, smallpox and yellow fever. While on America's East Coast blame for public health failures was directed towards the Irish, then the

Italians, and later towards Eastern European Jews, on the West Coast, any epidemic of infectious disease from smallpox to syphilis was blamed on the Chinese (Barde, 2003).

This discourse of blame resurfaced and was recontextualised in the case of SARS to fit contemporary political economic concerns, particularly around globalisation and the rise of the economic power of China. Yet how did the Chinese themselves respond to being blamed? NYC's Chinatown was stigmatised during the SARS epidemic, despite having no SARS cases, and people avoided the area and its restaurants. Research carried out with Chinese-American residents there revealed that many distanced themselves personally from risk, and instead identified their parents, children and the elderly as 'at risk'. At the same time they reaffirmed the association of Chinese culture with disease by redirecting blame onto recent Chinese immigrants, particularly those from Fujian Province, who had arrived illegally in the 1990s and represented a huge demographic shift within the NYC Chinese community. However, whether someone was regarded as a 'recent' immigrant was determined not by when they arrived, but by their degree of familiarity with American customs as opposed to their adherence to the customs of their country of origin, for example in respect of hygiene. In a demonstration of how people can be *othered* not just externally, but also within a community, Chinese New Yorkers spoke of the threat posed by recent immigrants, and overlaid this with notions of 'their' dangerous food, rural inferiority and alleged disregard for others (Eichelberger, 2007).

With the benefit of hindsight, SARS proved not to be 'the big one' that was feared at the time, although it is often cited as a 'rehearsal' for the threatened H5N1 influenza pandemic. In a Beckian sense, the risk moves elsewhere, always just over the horizon. In the end, SARS was contained through a combination of global surveillance, quarantine methods and travel bans. Despite talk of SARS being the 'first epidemic disease of the twenty-first century', SARS was contained by methods that would not have been unfamiliar to fourteenth-century Venetians. After 5 July there were no new cases reported, and on 14 July the WHO stopped publishing a daily table of the cumulative number of reported probable cases of SARS. In total, there had been a cumulative number of 8437 confirmed cases of SARS worldwide, of which 813 were fatal (World Health Organization, 2003a).

In sum, after the EID worldview gained wide currency in the middle of the 1990s, infectious diseases moved up the media and political agenda. Epidemics of new infectious diseases, or sometimes even the threat of epidemics, waxed and waned in the public(s) attention, with the pitch of the risk discourse ramped up with each new threat. The discourse surrounding these diseases is mapped onto *Risk Society* concerns in various ways: concerns about globalisation and the ease of modern travel and migration; about the economic interconnectedness of the globalised world; about the dissolving of the borders of the nation state; about the misuse of technology; and about the role of discredited and mistrusted expert opinion.

At the same time, we can discern at least two blaming patterns in the responses to EID. The first, seen in those diseases that affect 'people like us', such as 'superbugs' or (for the British at least) 'mad cow disease', directs the blame upwards to *our leaders*. The second, more usual blaming pattern distances the threat by *othering,* as seen in diseases that affect geographically distant or marginalised people, such as AIDS, Ebola and SARS. In Mary Douglas's terms, these patterns trace a connection between responses to the infectious diseases of late modernity and to more 'primitive' responses.

In both 'primitive' and modern responses to epidemics of infectious disease, a central and recurring *motif* is the hygiene of *others*, or more precisely their alleged lack of it. Thus, in the next chapter, it is to this delicate matter of personal hygiene, and to notions of dirt, germs and contagion, that we shall direct our attention.

6
Dirt, Germs and the Immune System

Thus far, the phenomenon of EID have been discussed in relation to the changes associated with late modernity, particularly concerns about globalisation and a heightened awareness of risk. As discussed in Chapter 4, the modern era began in Europe in the eighteenth century, with the advances in science and technology that accompanied the development of industrial capitalism. 'Modern' in this sense has a cluster of connotations relating to 'rational' and 'scientific'. Modern explanations of phenomena such as epidemics of infectious diseases ostensibly rely on rational evaluation of evidence gathered using scientific methods. 'Primitive' explanations of such phenomena, in contrast, rely on superstition or religious faith, and cast blame on individuals or groups by inventing causal connections between natural events and moral transgressions. This latter type of response is exemplified in allegations of witchcraft.

However, as discussed in Chapter 3, responses to AIDS in the 1980s, couched as they were in the language of accusation, racism and religious fundamentalism, hardly seemed very 'modern' in this sense. Alongside the apparently modern discourse around infectious disease there runs a parallel one, which links modern reactions to EID to more 'primitive' reactions to past plagues and pestilences. This chapter will explore how the way EID are conceptualised is influenced by pre-modern notions of dirt and contagion, and how such pre-bacteriological concepts are incorporated into more recent understandings of germs and the immune system.

Purity and Danger

In Chapter 4, there was a discussion of the English anthropologist Mary Douglas's later work on risk, in which she argues that despite being apparently based on rational science, modern responses to risk are little different to (what she calls) 'primitive' ones. The discussion of dirt here picks up another, earlier, strand of her work, in which she argues that ideas of purity and pollution are central to cultural life in modern, as well as in 'primitive', cultures.

In her ground-breaking book, *Purity and Danger,* Douglas (1966) examined religious purity rituals and prohibitions, which had previously been dismissed as irrational relics from a more superstitious past. For instance, in Chapter 11 of the Biblical book of Leviticus, there are a series of food prohibitions that make 'a difference between the unclean and the clean, and between the beast that may be eaten and the beast that may not be eaten.' To a modern reader, putting aside for a moment what we 'know' about germs, the assignation of certain things as *kosher* seems, on the face of it, completely random. For example, in Leviticus, locusts, beetles and grasshoppers are classified clean and therefore edible, as are animals that are cloven-footed *and* chew the cud. Swine are classified as unclean and inedible, because although they are cloven-footed, they do not chew the cud. Things that live in the water are classified as edible, so long as they have fins and scales, therefore shellfish, which have neither, are classified as an 'abomination'.

Douglas argues that, far from being random, these prohibitions rest on a system of classification. Things that do not 'fit' the orthodox classification are regarded as polluted because they cross or violate symbolic borders. 'Pollution' here is used not in the same sense that we might talk of a river being polluted, but in the sense of a contagious state, something harmful and mysterious, and caused by outside interference. For Douglas, pollution is therefore not simply the binary opposite of cleanliness, it arises out of a confusion of categories (Campkin, 2007).

The prohibition against eating shellfish thus has its roots in the classification of fish as creatures with scales. Shellfish are seen as violating the orthodox classification of 'fish' and thus are to be avoided as polluted. From a modern germ theory perspective, the prohibition against eating shellfish in the Middle East in the days before refrigeration makes perfect sense, simply as a means to avoid food poisoning. This is known as the 'medical materialist' perspective, which would argue that even the most apparently exotic of ancient rites must have a basis in hygiene. But, as Douglas points out, even if some of Moses' dietary rules were hygienically beneficial, this interpretation casts him as a sort of enlightened public health administrator, rather than a spiritual leader.

While she rejects medical materialist interpretations of the symbolic rituals and beliefs of 'primitive' peoples, Douglas also rejects the opposite view, which holds that there is nothing in common between modern ideas of cleanliness and 'primitive' rituals. For her, modern beliefs about dirt similarly express symbolic systems. The difference between pollution behaviours in different historical or anthropological contexts is only a matter of detail. However, there are two notable differences between ideas of dirt and defilement in modern and 'primitive' cultures. The first is that, for a modern European at least, the avoidance of dirt is not related to religion. The second is that modern ideas about dirt are dominated by knowledge of germs and the diseases they can cause, which stems from the advances in bacteriology since the 1880s.

Douglas thus argues that dirt has symbolic and metaphorical meanings beyond those offered by medical materialism and germ theory. As will be discussed in greater detail below, despite the differences between modern and 'primitive' notions of dirt, pre-bacteriological notions of contamination live on in the approach to dirt in modern thinking. Adapting Lord Palmerston's nineteenth-century phrase 'Dirt is matter in the wrong place', Douglas famously defined dirt as *matter out of place*. Dirt and pollution are thus socially constructed, and represent disorder, which must be restored by ordering and maintaining socially sanctioned boundaries between things considered clean and unclean.

Furthermore, as discussed in Chapter 4, this sense of spiritual purity and the danger of pollution becomes imprinted on a group, who use it to define who belongs within the group – who are 'people like us' – and who is classified as *other*. The perception of the dirtiness of *others*, whether they be 'the great unwashed' or 'smelly foreigners', thus reinforces dominant value systems and social boundaries (Campkin & Cox, 2007).

Douglas's later work picks up this theme and explores how and why *others* get blamed for misfortunes that affect the group, such as plagues. This 'primitive' pattern can be seen in responses to many EID discussed thus far: *others* are dirty/eat disgusting food/have bizarre rituals or customs/have perverted or promiscuous sex. Douglas demonstrated how fears of dirt and contamination become a source of social control, a weapon to exclude, thus exposing the moral dimensions that lie under the surface of even modern, apparently medical materialist, notions of cleanliness and dirt avoidance (Smith, 2007).

A quick and dirty history of personal hygiene

As Douglas points out, modern notions of dirt differ from 'primitive' ones in that they are dominated by germ theory and thus link dirt to germs and to infectious diseases. However, this understanding is only about 130 years old. How then did people understand dirt and its connection to disease before germ theory?

In Europe, from the time of the Roman Empire until around the eighteenth century, the body and disease were understood via the ancient Greek system of humourism. The humours were thought to be fluids within the body (black bile, yellow bile, phlegm and blood), with disease conceived as the result of an excess or deficiency of one of these fluids. Treatments such as bloodletting, emetics and purges were aimed at expelling a harmful surplus of a humour and thereby restoring equilibrium.

The word for the dirt that caused disease was *miasma,* from *miamo,* 'to pollute', via the root *mia,* meaning 'defilement' or 'destruction' (Smith, 2007). Miasmas were associated with foul airs resulting from decaying organic matter from cesspools, corpses and marshes, and exacerbated by extreme weather conditions. Although it was clear to contemporaries that plagues such as the Black Death were contagious, the cause of contagion was not conceptualised as a particle, but rather as a property of the air, which had been corrupted by miasmas.

As health was thought to rest on the correct balance of the humours, and because the body was regarded as permeable, over time immersion in water came to be thought of as dangerous to health. For Christians, the avoidance of washing also took on a spiritual dimension. The early Christians were of course Jews, with a heritage of Talmudic laws commanding cleanliness, or at least ritual purification. But by the fourth and fifth centuries Christians had come to regard dirtiness as a badge of holiness. This mortification of the flesh was known as *alousia,* 'the state of being unwashed', and was chosen by hermits, monks and saints, for whom any cleansing, except baptism, signified worldliness and vanity. This early Christian lack of concern about cleanliness is unusual among world religions: while the Spanish Christians washed neither their bodies nor clothes, Andalusian Arabs were known as 'the cleanest people on earth'. Damning evidence at the Spanish Inquisition, levelled at both Moors and Jews, was that the accused 'was known to bathe' (Ashenberg, 2007).

In the middle ages, people of all classes washed only rarely, believing that bathing could lead to possible exposure to pestilential air, as well as disrupt the humours. Consequently, most people were infested with vermin such as body lice, which they attributed to an excess of bodily humours. To control the humours, and thus the vermin, one's clothes could be changed, or at the very least kept clean. Over the centuries, the role of linen changed, and its regular renewal became a rule of cleanliness. Wiping was regarded as being the same as washing. Fresh white linen was thought to remove dirt by its intimate contact with the body, an effect surer and less dangerous than that of water (Vigarello, 1988).

Miasmic theory also held that stenches could be inhaled and incorporated into the body, thus affecting an individual's odour or appearance. So, for example, excessive indulgence in coitus was thought to provoke an overflow of semen into a woman's humours. Prostitutes were thus said to stink, and were considered dangerous sources of contamination. It was claimed that Jews emitted the *foetor judaicus*, a sulphuric smell believed to be the cause of illness and death, which was said to disappear on conversion to Christianity (Nelkin & Gilman, 1988).

Miasmas were conveyed particularly by the breath and body odours; the foul smell of hospitals was thought to be caused by the patients' quickened respiration, sweat, pus and sputum, from which the effluvia of disease emerged. Infection could be avoided, and resistance to it increased, by wearing strong perfume or burning sweet-smelling pellets in a perfume pan. Such fumigants were thought to be capable of destroying the presence of plague in bodies, fabrics and clothing.

Apart from aromatics, the other tactic to destroy miasmas was ventilation. Pure air was thought to be the best antiseptic, and disinfection consisted of ventilation, draining off refuse and preventing individuals from crowding together (Corbin, 1986). This view remained current even in the time of Florence Nightingale, who held the germ theory of disease in contempt, and whose reforms of hospital sanitation during the Crimean War in the 1850s were based on her belief in dispelling miasmas with pure air.

Before the middle of the eighteenth century, correcting body odour through the application of perfume was also held to purify. Thereafter, the use of heavy perfumes gradually began to fall out of fashion, as perfume was said only to disguise putrid miasmas. Instead, attention began to be focused on the purity and healthiness of the air (Vigarello, 1988). The threshold of tolerance to smell suddenly lowered, at least amongst the elite, and odours began to be more keenly smelled. By the end of the eighteenth century, even the masses had this new sensibility, especially with regard to the smell of excrement (Corbin, 1986).

Around the end of the eighteenth century, it became fashionable for the upper classes to have baths and bathrooms in their homes, although their purpose was luxury rather than cleanliness. At around this time, the notion also arose that a cold bath produced vigour and resistance, and was beneficial to health. For the first time, bathing came to have an explicitly hygienic role, not because it washed, but because it *strength-ened*. The contrast was drawn between the character-building ordeal of the cold bath, and the enfeebling, effeminising luxury of the warm bath. Ideas about cold baths also intersected with the contemporary introduc-tion of smallpox inoculation, which, like the cold bath, was thought to strengthen by operating on a supposed underlying resistance to illness (Vigarello, 1988).

In the early nineteenth century, the idea of the skin's respiratory func-tion captured the attention of scientists on both sides of the Atlantic. It was proposed that if pores were clogged with dirt then carbon diox-ide could not exit through the skin (Ashenberg, 2007). Soap now began to be used for washing, and began to be regarded as a tool of health rather than an elegant luxury. Although miasmic explanations were still dominant, by the time of the 1832 'Asiatic' cholera epidemic in Europe, water now came to be seen as playing a protective role against disease, a dramatic reversal since the time of the Black Death. As discussed in Chapter 2, the terror of cholera, associated with the overcrowding, poor sanitation and filth of the nineteenth century urban slums led to cam-paigns to eradicate disease and cleanse the cities of their filth. These were at once vast improvements and often violently discriminatory, dove-tailing with the increasing state regulation of individuals' bodies and freedoms, particularly in relation to the poor (Cohen, 2005).

References to the stenches arising from the earth, stagnant water, corpses and carcasses diminished in the nineteenth century, and instead there was a growing obsession with the odours of poverty. Up to this point there had been a rough equality between the classes in terms of their smell. A new kind of distinction now arose between the classes. The absence of an intrusive odour enabled the individual to distinguish himself from 'the great unwashed', a term coined by Thackeray in 1849. Whereas in the eighteenth century the odour of bodies was connected with the climate, diet, profession and temperament, the new attitude connected odours to the poor (Corbin, 1986). Servants and working men smelled unpleasant, an attitude neatly summed up by George Orwell in *The Road to Wigan Pier:* 'The lower classes smell'.

Although William Budd and John Snow had proposed a theory of disease based on bacteria as early as 1849, their views failed to gain widespread acceptance. By the middle of the nineteenth century, European and American doctors had split into two broad camps: the sanitarians, or hygienists, who clung to the idea of miasmas; and the contagionists, who advocated germ theory (Sachs, 2007). Pasteur's *Germ Theory and its Application to Medicine* was published in 1861, but it took a long time for germ theory to gain the upper hand. For a while, some believed in both germs and miasmas, as the new concept of germs fitted easily into older popular notions of living particles – *contagium vivum.* However, it was Koch's discovery of specificity, that each germ was a separate species with a life of its own, that ultimately undermined the miasmic theory of the sanitarians (Smith, 2007). By the 1880s Pasteur's and Koch's discoveries had become predominant, marking the end of the belief in miasmas amongst scientists, and with it the link between smells and contagion.

Germs, hygiene and the immune system

The new science of bacteriology transformed the concept of dirt and the hygiene practices associated with it. Henceforth, families were said to need bathrooms in the war against germs. Providing baths for the working classes was seen as an important means of reducing the spread of infectious diseases across all strata of society. Soap producers funded campaigns to spread 'good' habits such as hand washing before eating and after going to the toilet. By 1938, a survey showed that soap ranked second only to bread and butter as one of life's essentials (Shove, 2003).

Although the word 'contagious' was dropped from medical discourse around 1910 (when the official US Public Health Handbook of Infectious Diseases first substituted the term 'communicable'), the older concept of contagion became elided with the new bacteriological concept of germs. Contagion located the source of disease as outside the body, in other people, the air they had breathed or the surfaces they had touched. Ideas and practices associated with the fear of contagion through contact with other people's germs were a vital lesson of childhood acculturation in Western societies in the early twentieth century. Children, or middle-class children at least, were warned of the dangers of germs from putting things in their mouths, and were instructed to wash their hands before eating (Pernick, 2002).

Another aspect of the concept of contagion was the emphasis on the danger of 'close contact', particularly sexual contact. An example of the dread of contagion, and of its links to sexual morality was what has been called 'syphilophobia'. In early twentieth-century America, there was a widespread belief that syphilis could be contracted through the brief contacts of everyday life – at the grocery, in the park, at the barber shop, or from toilet seats (the fear of infected toilet seats resurfaced in the late 1980s with regards to AIDS). The concern was that 'immorally' contracted syphilis would be then passed to native, middle-class 'moral' Americans. The interest in 'venereal disease' was further heightened during both world wars, with the compulsory examination and incarceration of thousands of women suspected of prostitution or 'promiscuity' – a 'promiscuous man' considered oxymoronic. Despite campaigns emphasising that venereal disease affected all sections of society, the view persisted that certain groups, such as ethnic minorities and the working class, were particularly affected and therefore to blame (Brandt, 1985).

By the 1940s and 1950s, the most important defence against the germs lurking in the environment just outside the body was by preventing their entrance into the body through cleanliness, washing and personal habits, such as not touching the mouth with the hands. American women's magazines of the period depicted the body as a castle, with mothers/women keeping the invading germs outside the castle walls through cleaning. Poliomyelitis epidemics in the 1950s led popular periodicals to turn their attention to defences *within* the body. By the 1960s and 1970s, the newly popularised concept of the immune response was as a single interconnected *system,* residing entirely inside the body. This notion led to a diminishing concern with hygiene and the cleanliness of the outer surfaces of the body (Martin, 1994).

It has been argued that the dominance of the military metaphor used in relation to infectious disease arose as a result of the coincidence of the emergence of germ theory from France in the 1860s and 1870s with the threat posed to France at that time by Prussian militarisation. Given that cultural milieu, the germs that caused disease came to be conceptualised as evil invaders. The military metaphor subsequently became the dominant way of understanding twentieth-century medicine, portraying diseases and the germs that caused them as enemies in a modern war, a threatening, alien *other* (Gwyn, 1999).

The appearance of AIDS in the 1980s led to an enormously increased interest in the immune system in both scientific and lay audiences. The HIV virus was understood as destroying the body's defences from the inside of the very cells responsible for its defence (Moulin, 2000). In her essay *AIDS and its Metaphors,* Susan Sontag (1989) argued that while the early AIDS epidemic had been dominated by the 'gay plague' metaphor, the middle of the 1980s saw a new set of metaphors come into play. These built on the military metaphors common in bacteriology, but also reflected the age of *Star Wars* and *Space Invaders,* as well as the dawning information age. Thus by a process of repeated exposure to certain metaphors it became natural to talk of the HIV virus *docking* onto the

T-cell, *reprogramming* the cell to produce more HIV and *hijacking* the body's own *defences*.

In the years following the appearance of AIDS, the immune system became central to Western scientific and lay conceptions of health. People were exhorted to 'strengthen' their immune system by attention to diet and by minimising stress, and thus to transform or train their immune system and render it superior (Martin, 1994). This way of conceptualising the immune system became embedded into representations of health and infectious diseases and, as discussed below, became particularly pertinent, for example, in the discourse around 'superbugs' in the late 1990s.

Although rooted in scientific notions, ironically the notion of the immune system as something that individuals can 'bolster' also transected with the growth of interest in the 'alternative' medicine movement, which saw an astonishing rise in popularity from the 1980s onwards. By 2005 alternative medicine was used by around half of the population of European countries such as France, Belgium, Germany and Denmark, and by up to 70 per cent of people in Australia, America and Canada. In 2005, one in ten people visited one of the estimated 47,000 alternative practitioners in Britain, compared to 35,000 medical General Practitioners (Shapiro, 2008).

Alternative approaches to health are often based on 'holistic' notions of disease being caused by a weakened immune system. Contaminants in the environment, such as 'junk' food or air pollution, are said to damage the immune system, as are conventional medical treatments, such as those for cancer or AIDS. The immune system is then understood to need support by various supplements and through special diets. This approach is rooted in the notion that we are individually responsible for our own health, and through self-help methods can wrest control of our bodies away from both the disease itself and from a 'biomedical model', which is regarded as alienating. Whilst alternative medicine is dismissed by most of the medical establishment as quackery, and as a softer form of victim blaming, its widespread popularity suggests both a loss of faith in conventional 'scientific' medicine and that its underpinning conception of the immune system has deep cultural resonance.

America saw a renewed emphasis on the invisible dangers lurking from germs in the light of the so-called 'war on terror'. A 2006 article in *The New York Times* reported on a range of new consumer products reaching the US market, including: *Purell-2-Go*, a hand-sanitising gel manufactured by the pharmaceutical giant Pfizer, which came in small bottles with rubber rings to attach it to backpacks, lunchboxes and key chains ('We tried to make it fun', gushed a Pfizer spokeswoman); *Safe-T-Gard*, 'a combination dispenser of doorknob-sized tissues and trash receptacle' to be mounted on the wall next to public toilet doors; *Sanit-Grasp*, a U-shaped handle which allowed toilet cubicle doors to be opened using the forearm; a portable subway strap that promised to do away with 'reaching for a slimy overhead bar'; ultraviolet 'pens' that could be dipped into a glass of water to kill DNA; and an air purifier to be worn around the neck as a pendant. Echoing the importance placed on hand hygiene a century earlier, an American children's book published in 2005 called *Germs are Not for Sharing* instructed: 'When germs get on your hands, they can spread to other people... [w]hen you hold hands or play games or give each other high fives' (Salkin, 2006).

It is easy to lampoon American germ phobia as related to a sense of loss of control in a threatening post-9/11 world. Yet a similar renewed focus on the transmission of germs, particularly through poor hand hygiene, also pervaded the British media coverage of the 'superbug' MRSA. As discussed in the previous chapter, the British media and political discourse around MRSA was dominated by descriptions of dirty hospitals. An apparently modern discussion of the danger of dirt (because of the pathogenicity of bacteria) obscured a more fundamental and 'primitive' fear of an invisible danger lurking in the chaos of underfunded and poorly managed hospitals (Washer & Joffe, 2006).

Research carried out with a cross-section of the British public found that these media representations of MRSA were widely shared by the audience, as was the perceived solution of improved hospital hygiene, enforced by the return of the matron. Yet while scientific/biomedical accounts of MRSA would, at least in part, blame the emergence of antibiotic-resistant strains of bacteria on the overprescription of antibiotics, only a minority of the respondents in this research (the broadsheet-reading men) made any link between MRSA and antibiotic use. The distinction between healthy self and diseased *other* was transformed in the lay discourse around MRSA. Lay notions of the immune system led to a new distinction being made between the invulnerable healthy self with a 'boosted immune system' and the diseased immunocompromised *other*, such as the elderly or those already hospitalised. As with othering mechanisms seen in relation to responses to other EID such as AIDS, the distinction served the same function, which was to distance the perceived threat of MRSA from the self and project it onto *others* perceived to be at risk (Washer et al., 2008).

One of the difficulties in trying to disentangle those practices associated with modern germ avoidance from those which have their roots in more 'primitive' notions of contagion lies in distinguishing those practices where we 'know' that the reason for the dirt avoidance practice is to protect against contracting an infection. It is easier to pin-point more 'primitive' notions of contagion within 'modern' practices in contexts other than those involving infectious diseases, where there are no germs which could contaminate, yet still people have practices that symbolically separate the healthy self from the contaminating *other*.

One such example is Jodelet's (1991) fascinating study of an open psychiatric institution in central France in the 1970s, where for several generations mentally ill patients had been placed in the care of local families. One of the most striking behaviours in the vast majority of placements was the families' separation of the lodgers' cutlery, crockery, glasses, and sometimes even laundry. The families themselves had difficulty accounting for these practices. Although they denied the possibility of contagion with the mental illness of the lodgers (in the medical sense), they still evidenced fear of some sort of 'magical' contagion.

This example of the separation of the lodgers' from the families' cutlery, crockery and glasses is a contagion practice that persisted even when it was accepted there were no 'germs' to catch. As Norbert Elias (1939) points out in *The History of Manners*, although we take individual cutlery entirely for granted, even as late as the seventeenth century in Europe the fork was a luxury item for the upper classes only, usually made of gold or silver. Before that, in the medieval period, everyone ate from the same dish with their hands. A medical materialist explanation might see the elimination of eating with the hands, the introduction of the fork, individual cutlery and crockery, and all other modern Western food rituals as being based on 'hygienic grounds'. But even as late as the second half of the eighteenth century there is hardly any evidence for that kind of motivation.

There is nothing to suggest that changes in manners came about for reasons that were 'rational' or were related to causal connections to health. The delicacy of feeling demonstrated through developments in Western table manners were only later justified through scientific understandings of hygiene. Modern sensibility is that it is unhygienic to eat with the fingers because of contact with the germs of others, who may be diseased. Yet, as Elias points out, to take bread or cake from one's own plate and put it into our mouths with our fingers is no more hygienic. Most of what we call 'hygiene' thus has the same function as 'morality', which is to condition children to a certain standard of socially desirable behaviour, even though it may appear that that behaviour is in the interests of health or human dignity.

As discussed in the previous chapter, in the Western media coverage of the SARS epidemic, one of the ways in which the Chinese were *othered* was through attention to their alleged poor hygiene, in particular the practice of spitting in public places. The media descriptions of such practices are clearly meant to invoke 'our' disgust at the way 'they' behave. Take this example of a report of a Chinese market during the height of the SARS panic, from a liberal British broadsheet, the *Independent on Sunday*:

> ...As I watched a man buying scorpions, the woman serving him hawked a gob of sputum from her throat, lurched to her feet and spat expertly behind my heel. Spitting is as natural as sneezing here – bubbles of phlegm pepper the streets – and could be spreading the virus. Of such simple habits are global epidemics made. (Laurance, 2003)

European squeamishness around spitting in public thus confirms the superiority of Western civilisation. Yet even in Europe, spitting in public was not only common amongst all classes until relatively recently, but was also felt to be necessary. Only through the seventeenth and eighteenth centuries did the practice become more and more distasteful, until it came to be considered shameful. Like the example of the use of cutlery to eat, this change in behaviour was driven by rising societal thresholds of repugnance, rather than by a medical materialist understanding of germs and their transmission through sputum (Elias, 1939).

As discussed above, miasmic theory connected unpleasant smells with the sources of contagion and held that prophylaxis against disease was achieved by removing the smell, either by disguising it with aromatics or perfume or through ventilation. The acceptance of germ theory severed the connection that had previously existed between smell and disease. Over the past 100 years or so, the importance of smell has become increasingly marginalised in Western culture. Darwin, in *The Descent of Man,* postulated that humans lost their acuity of smell in the process of evolving from animals. Freud, in *Civilization and its Discontents,* held that smell had given way to sight when the human species began to walk upright, removing the nose from the proximity of scent trails and increasing the visual field (Classen et al., 1994). In the modern world, or the developed world at least, smell is mostly noticeable by its absence.

However, smell still connects modern understandings of germs to a more 'primitive' miasmic fear of contagion. For example, a recurring *motif* of the British media's coverage of MRSA, as well as in the audience responses to that coverage were lurid descriptions of toilets, bodily functions and their association with particular smells. These were contrasted with the antiseptic 'hospital' smell associated with the 'spotless', 'pristine' wards which the matron would enforce. The lack of a foul smell and/or the presence of a disinfectant smell in a hospital thus suggested to people that infection had been dealt with. This olfactory reassurance is in fact mistaken – disinfectant solutions are often used inappropriately and have been shown to be the sources of contamination and infections in hospitals (Ayliffe & English, 2003).

Be that as it may, the accounts of smells associated with 'superbugs' reveal traces of a cultural residue of pre-scientific conceptions of contagion, located within and alongside a framework of modern scientific understandings.

The hygiene hypothesis

Throughout the twentieth century in Western societies, levels of expected cleanliness both escalated and became standardised. For example, the daily shower came to replace the once traditional weekly bath, and an expectation arose that freshly laundered clothes should be worn each day. Conventions of cleanliness in contemporary Western societies demanded increasingly frequent washing, despite the decrease in environmental dirt arising from developments such as mains water and sewerage systems, paved streets, the use of cars rather than horses as transport, the introduction of electric power and decreasing dependence on coal (Shove, 2003).

Thus far, the narrative has been of a notion of 'progress' towards ever 'higher' standards of hygiene, by which is usually meant Euro-American standards of washing and disinfection. However, this increase in cleanliness has led to another recent strand of the discourse around dirt, which argues that 'we' are now *too clean,* and that rather than preventing diseases, this over-cleanliness is causing disease.

Over the past few generations, more affluent, Western countries have seen an enormous increase in autoimmune diseases such as Type 1 diabetes, Crohn's disease and multiple sclerosis, as well as of allergic diseases such as asthma, allergic rhinitis and atopic dermatitis. Whilst there is a familial element to allergies and asthma, it is nevertheless clear that their prevalence has increased: in some developed countries up to 40 per cent of children have asthma. There is also evidently some link between Western 'lifestyle' and allergic diseases. For example, recent immigrants from the developing world often develop allergies around five years after immigration to the developed world; and after German reunification the previously lower prevalence of allergies in East Germany rose to the same, higher, prevalence as in West Germany (Kaufmann, 2009).

In 1989, Strachan first proposed the so-called 'hygiene hypothesis'. He showed that the prevalence of hay fever in British children, which had been increasing for 30 years, was inversely related to the number of children in the household. He suggested that unhygienic contact with older siblings led to infections with viral illnesses, particularly of the respiratory tract, such as the common cold, measles, mumps and rubella, and that this exposure conferred protection against hay fever. Thus he proposed that in wealthier countries declining family size, improvements in household amenities, and higher standards of personal cleanliness were responsible for a reduced opportunity for cross-infection in young families and a resulting rise in allergic disease such as hay fever (Strachan, 1989).

Since first proposed, evidence has accumulated to support the 'hygiene hypothesis'. For example, epidemiological studies of Italian Air Force personnel found that respiratory allergy was less frequent in those people heavily exposed to food-borne microbes transmitted via the faecal–oral route, such as *Toxoplasma gondii* and *Helicobacter pylori*. This suggests that hygiene and a Westernised semi-sterile diet may stimulate the tendency to develop allergies by influencing the overall pattern of pathogens that stimulate the gut, thus contributing to the epidemic of allergic asthma and rhinitis in developed countries. Such data support the hypothesis that allergies may be prevented by eating traditionally processed food, not treated with antimicrobial preservatives and not subjected to hygienic procedures (Matricardi et al., 2000).

Later studies have proposed that protection against allergies is not endowed by childhood viral illnesses but rather by early and continual exposure to non-disease-causing microbes, especially the kind that children come into contact with around other children and animals. For example, children growing up on farms are exposed to a greater diversity of microbes, yet have a lower prevalence of allergies compared to neighbouring children not brought up on farms but from the same villages. This indicates that even when there is no apparent illness an immune response is stimulated which protects against allergies, and, conversely, the lack of such exposure seems to promote immune disorders in people with an underlying predisposition for them. The suggestion is that harmless 'colonisation' by environmental bacteria that pass through the body acts as an immune regulator (Sachs, 2007; Schaub et al., 2006).

This new conceptualisation of the relationship between people and germs has led some to be concerned about the potential harm that antibiotics may cause, as they kill normal 'good germs' in the gut. A number of studies have found an association between antibiotic use in children and asthma, although this may be because in many countries children with asthma are likely to have been inappropriately prescribed antibiotics (Sachs, 2007; Schaub et al., 2006).

The popularisation of the notion of 'good bacteria' associated with the hygiene hypothesis has led to the launch of 'probiotic' supplements added to yoghurts, which have become one of the fastest-growing sectors of the dairy market, despite their benefit to healthy people being uncertain. Probiotics have an ambivalent status, being marketed as science-based products and yet also advocated as an advance in alternative medicine. Their official advertising, which is subject to advertising standards regulation, claims only that they 'maintain digestive health' by 'improving digestive transit'. However, media coverage claims that they can prevent infectious diseases, improve thinning hair, even prevent autism. The ills of modernity, such as improper diets, stress and lack of energy are said to be particularly susceptible to 'treatment' with probiotics. The media coverage of probiotics does not question the assumption that we need to 'top up' our 'good bacteria'. Consumers seem to be increasingly buying into the promise that probiotics can rebalance an inner order in a risky and disorderly outer world (Nerlich & Koteyko, 2008).

The return of the anti-vaccination movement

As well as concerns about modern attitudes to hygiene harming the immune system by not stimulating it enough, another related strand of the contemporary discourse around the immune system and infectious diseases argues that negative health consequences follow from *overstimulation* of the immune system through vaccination.

Modern Western anti-vaccination movements have inherited some of the nineteenth-century anti-vaccination libertarian rhetoric (as discussed in Chapter 2), although not the religious interpretation of vaccination as interfering with God's will. Instead, parents in the developed world now often conceptualise vaccination as 'interfering with nature'. The modern anti-vaccination debate started in the 1970s, with concerns in Britain that pertussis (whooping cough) vaccination was linked to brain damage. As a result, pertussis vaccination coverage fell from around 70 to 80 per cent to around 40 per cent of British children. In 1979, the British government introduced a Vaccine Damage Payment Act and confidence in pertussis vaccination was gradually restored.

The 1980s and 1990s saw new anti-vaccination groups emerge in many Western societies, facilitated by the then novel technology of the Internet. These groups were often associated with the advocacy of alternative medicine and made a range of claims about the harm said to be associated with vaccinations. They argued that the diseases were anyway declining, that vaccines were a violation of civil liberties, that adverse events were under-reported, that vaccines caused idiopathic illness and that they eroded immunity, and that vaccine policy was motivated by profit and promoted by 'big pharma' (Blume, 2006).

In 1998, a study published in the medical journal *The Lancet* reported data from 12 children suggesting a possible temporal association between the measles, mumps and rubella vaccine (MMR) and the development of inflammatory bowel disease and autism (Wakefield et al., 1998). The resulting furore led to MMR vaccination rates dropping to a record low in the UK. Falls in MMR coverage were reported in other northern European countries, the USA, Australia and New Zealand, although though not to the same extent as in Britain. The research in question was independently reviewed several times, and scientific opinion very strongly refuted the suggestion of any link between MMR and autism. The paper was later retracted, and the study's author, Dr Andrew Wakefield, was charged with professional misconduct.

It has been suggested that the MMR controversy had greater resonance in Britain because it came so soon after the BSE episode there. Journalists and the public alike were suspicious of government and health officials and questioned expert opinion (Singh et al., 2007). The confidence of British parents was also shaken by the refusal of the prime minister, Tony Blair, despite relentless media speculation, to confirm or deny whether his own infant son had received the vaccination. As a result of poor MMR coverage, in 2006, Britain had an epidemic of measles, with 300 cases, the largest outbreak since the introduction of the MMR vaccine at the end of the 1980s.

Similar anti-vaccination sentiments found fertile ground in the Netherlands and in Germany, where as a result of declining vaccination coverage 17 children and adolescents died from complications of measles between 2003 and 2007 (Kaufmann, 2009). Research in the Netherlands found parents who were opposed to vaccination were well educated but resisted (particularly the measles) vaccination on the grounds that they were convinced that it could impair the immune system, or that vaccinations in general had long-term and unknown side-effects. Their decisions were sometimes based on assumptions about the learning capacity of the immune system. Parents believed in keeping the immune system 'strong' through the use of alternative medicine (Streefland et al., 1999).

A study of English parents regarding their MMR decisions also found that more experience of alternative medicine correlated with rejection of the MMR, although not all parents who used alternative therapies refused to vaccinate, and conversely not all non-vaccinators embraced alternative therapies. In light of the proposed link between the BSE and MMR controversies made above, parents in this study seldom mentioned the controversy over BSE as influencing their lack of trust over MMR, and a few actively denied that the BSE controversy had influenced their views on MMR. They tended to conceptualise their child's health as shaped by family history, birth and other illnesses, and they incorporated concerns about sleep, allergies, dietary tolerances, character and behaviour as all influencing a child's particular vulnerabilities to disease or vaccination. Parents reflected not on 'risks' or 'safety' in general, but whether they thought the vaccination was right for *their* child (Poltorak et al., 2005).

The re-emergence of anti-vaccination movements echoes some aspects of Giddens's conception of late modern societies, as discussed in Chapter 4. The new anti-vaccination movement is facilitated by one of the features of the globalised late modern society, namely the mass media and the Internet. The movement also links to Giddens's conception of the reflexivity of late modernity, and reflects the detraditionalisation of society. In earlier societies the pronouncements of 'experts' (in religion, science or medicine) provided secure 'knowledge' that people were expected to follow. However, in late modern societies growing numbers of parents are beset by doubt about the risks of vaccination, and question expert opinion.

This speaks to the changing relationship with 'expert' knowledge and lack of trust in the institutions of modernity, including medicine, the media and government. Potential risks, such as those felt to arise from vaccinations, are reflexively examined by individual parents. Risks are then framed as relating to *their* particular child's health and in relation to new constantly incoming scientific and lay 'knowledge' about the risk of vaccination. The critical stance against vaccination is a logical consequence of the wresting of control away from medical 'experts' and the shift towards consumerism, informed choice and empowerment in health, in light of which educated Western patients and parents also expect to make informed choices in other areas, for example in the rise of the natural childbirth movement (Blume, 2006).

This discussion of the MMR here also links with Beck's *Risk Society* thesis. The risks said to arise from vaccinations, do not occur 'naturally' but are a product of medical intervention. At the same time it is scientists and medical 'experts' themselves who judge the safety of vaccinations. The MMR scare captures many of the features the *Risk Society*. Anti-vaccinationists hold that the chains of cause and effect to the alleged vaccination adverse events are difficult or impossible to trace. Although MMR is most often thought to lead to immediate harm by causing autism soon after administration of the vaccine, some anti-vaccinationists have argued that the risk has a potentially long latency period and allege long-term reactions to vaccines due to them damaging the immune system (Dew, 1999). The risk of MMR vaccination is also said by its opponents to be incalculable, its consequences impossible to estimate scientifically. MMR also seems to fit the Beckian model insofar that the consequences of MMR – allegedly autism – may be so catastrophic that no amount of compensation would offset the risk.

The growth in interest in alternative medicine, with its roots in the scientific conception of the immune system, and its association with the modern anti-vaccination movement also speaks to a new relationship between the ideas of dirt, germs and health in late modern society. The 'hygiene hypothesis' brings us back to Douglas's idea that dirt as *matter out of place*. Germs are now recast, not as negatively associated with dirt, but as necessary. 'Good germs' *in the right place* are seen as essential for the maintenance of health, by 'testing' and 'strengthening' the immune system. This definition of 'good germs' includes respiratory viruses, pathogens from farm animals, even food-borne microbes transmitted via the faecal–oral route.

A century ago, the new germ theory perceived the avoidance of other people's germs through strict hand washing and other hygiene practices as essential for the maintenance of health. In this new understanding, the germ phobia that leads Americans to avoid touching handrails on public transport is now portrayed as damaging their immune systems and thus their health. 'Good germs' are recast as necessary for the avoidance of an epidemic of diseases of the immune system that are associated with modernity. The immune system is understood as needing to 'learn from the environment' in order to function correctly. Thus the hygiene hypothesis links to the notion that the 're-emergence' of infectious diseases is in part linked to modernity, and to ideas about the 'unnatural' semi-sterile processed foods and of 'harmful' antibiotics, which are now no longer thought of as 'magic bullets', because they alter the 'natural' 'good' bacteria in the human gut (Rook & Stanford, 1998).

The discussion of changing conceptions of dirt to something seen as in some sense 'good for us', brings us back to Douglas's notion that modern beliefs about dirt express symbolic systems and have metaphorical meanings beyond those offered by medical materialism and germ theory. One of the sources of resistance to vaccination lies in the sense of dread of contamination of a clean, pure, healthy body, particularly of a baby (Spier, 2002). Instead of vaccinations protecting against contaminating germs, this new social construction incorporates medical materialist notions of cleanliness and pollution with a cluster of lay understandings of the role of dirt, of hygiene, germs and the immune system. This worldview perceives non-vaccination as restoring the 'natural' order of things. It is not so much that modern notions of dirt and germs have replaced 'primitive' ones, nor has the pendulum swung back in some way in the light of the 'hygiene hypothesis' to pre-modern conceptions of cleanliness. Rather, the discussion in this chapter points to the conclusion that 'primitive' pre-bacteriological conceptions of dirt and its relationship to contagion coexist with biomedical notions.

While concerns about damage to the immune system and threats from naturally occurring epidemics grew through the 1990s, another different strand of the discourse around germs, contamination and containment gradually came into view. The next chapter will explore how, in parallel to the EID discourse, a new threat garnered increasing attention. This new discourse used much of the same language, metaphors and concepts as those used around EID, and the solutions to both problems were said to be shared. The next chapter will explore how the EID discourse was metaphorically hijacked by the newly emerging discourse around bioterrorism.

7
The Bioterrorism Myth

In the 1990s, a new microbial threat to America began to occupy the minds of the US government and its policy makers, and would eventually be filtered into the public consciousness by the mass media. The anthrax letters bioterrorism attacks of 2001 were by no means an unexpected event: America had been preparing for such an eventuality for over ten years. This chapter will explore how the discourse around bioterrorism became threaded through the discourse around EID. The cast of actors involved in promoting and popularising the threat from bioterrorists contained many of the same scientists, public health officials and writers as had promoted the EID worldview. The bioterrorism and the EID scripts were also very similar, in that both aimed to increase attention and funding given to the neglected US public health system.

The 2001 anthrax letters

On 18 September 2001, exactly one week after the 9/11 terrorist attacks, five letters were posted in standard pre-stamped US Postal Service issue envelopes from Trenton, New Jersey. Four of the letters were addressed to New York-based media: to ABC, to CBS, one to NBC news anchor Tom Brokaw and to the editor of the *New York Post*. One letter was addressed to the office of the tabloid the *National Enquirer* in Boca Raton, Florida. Three weeks later, on 9 October, two more letters were posted to Democratic senators in Washington DC, one addressed to Senator Tom Daschle and the other to Senator Patrick Leahy. The envelopes all contained a letter with statements such as '09-11-01. You cannot stop us. We have this anthrax. You die now. Are you afraid? Death to America. Death to Israel. Allah is great'. Each of the envelopes also contained powdered anthrax.

Anthrax (*Bacillus anthracis*) is a bacterium commonly seen in grazing animals, and can result in the sudden death of an infected animal. Bodily fluids from the carcass containing anthrax bacteria can then leak into the soil where they assume a protective spore form that can persist for as long as 70 years. Although anthrax rarely infects humans, spores can enter the body through a cut in the skin and cause cutaneous anthrax. Without antibiotic treatment the fatality rate from cutaneous anthrax can be 20 per cent, although with appropriate antibiotics this would be reduced to closer to 5 per cent. Rarer, but more dangerous, with a fatality rate of between 25 and 100 per cent, is gastrointestinal anthrax, caused through eating infected and undercooked meat. This sometimes occurs in developing countries, or where animals are not vaccinated or inspected. Very rarely, the spores can be breathed into the lungs causing inhalation anthrax. In both gastrointestinal and inhalation anthrax, the bacteria produce a toxin that can cause shock and pneumonia. Although antibiotics can be used to combat the infection, it is still difficult to treat, and untreated inhalation anthrax is almost inevitably fatal (Guillemin, 1999).

Approximately four days after the 18 September envelopes were mailed, a cluster of nine cases of anthrax infection emerged, with a second cluster of cases following approximately five days after the 9 October envelopes were mailed. In all, 22 people were infected, 11 with cutaneous anthrax and 11 with inhalation anthrax, of which five died. Illness and death occurred not only at the targeted workplaces, but also along the path of the mail and in other settings, and 20 of those infected were either mail handlers or were exposed at workplaces where contaminated mail was processed or received (Jernigan et al., 2002).

In the resulting panic, prescriptions for the powerful antibiotic ciprofloxacin – 'Cipro' – usually kept as a last resort when all other antibiotics have failed, increased by 42 per cent across the USA and by 203 per cent in the New York area (Trotter, 2003). More than 30,000 people in the USA are estimated to have received prophylactic antibiotics as a consequence of possible or suspected exposure to anthrax spores (Lane & Fauci, 2001). Ciprofloxacin is one of the class of quinolone antibiotics, which were all threatened with being compromised by this overuse with the development of antibiotic resistance (Shnayerson & Plotkin, 2002).

From very early in the investigation, the US Federal Bureau of Investigation (FBI) suspected that the powdered anthrax used in the letters was evidence of sophisticated 'weapons grade' technology: the powder was electro-statically charged and treated with silicon nano-particles as well as polymerised glass, materials not previously encountered in this connection (Matsumoto, 2003). (The claim that the anthrax contained sophisticated silicon additives was later disputed by scientists who argued that the silicon was encapsulated within the spores and thus naturally occurring (Bhattacharjee, 2008).)

The silicon prevented the natural tendency for the spores to form 'clumps', and instead allowed them to float freely in the air when the envelopes were opened, thus making them more dangerous, as they were more likely to be inhaled. This danger was not fully communicated, as the FBI would not share its samples with the CDC, which meant that health officials had to rely on the FBI's (false) reassurances that spores could not escape from envelopes (Clarke et al., 2006).

Initially, the FBI promoted the idea that a low-budget amateur could have produced this weaponised form of anthrax powder, although this 'do-it-yourself' anthrax scenario lost credibility when the FBI failed to engineer such a high-quality anthrax powder using basic equipment (Matsumoto, 2003). Analysis of the strain and properties of the anthrax used in the attacks soon indicated that it originated from within the US biodefence programme. In a paper published in the journal *Science,* researchers identified the strain of anthrax used in the letters as one that had originally come from a US military laboratory (Read et al., 2002). A *New Scientist* journalist revealed that the attack strain most likely originated from United States Army Medical Research Institute for Infectious Diseases (USAMRIID) laboratories. According to military sources, the US Army had been experimenting with various brands of silica nano-particles to add to germ warfare powders (Matsumoto, 2003).

In August 2002, the US Attorney General John Ashcroft revealed that investigators at the Justice Department had identified a so-called 'person of interest', Dr Steven J. Hatfill, a virologist who had worked on Ebola at the USAMRIID facility in Fort Detrick, Maryland in 1997. Hatfill vigorously denied responsibility and sued the US government. In 2008, the government paid him US$4.6 million in a without prejudice out-of-court settlement.

In July 2008, Dr Bruce Ivins, another former government scientist at Fort Detrick, apparently committed suicide after learning that the FBI were preparing a prosecution case against him for the anthrax attacks. The FBI later claimed that Ivins was solely responsible for the attacks, although that claim has been met with widespread scepticism, in part because Ivins seemed to lack a motive, and also because no evidence could be found placing him in New Jersey on any of the days the envelopes were mailed (Enserink, 2008).

Bioterror in history

The use, or alleged use, of infectious diseases as weapons to terrorise one's enemies has a long history. The earliest accounts of infectious diseases apparently used to deliberately infect an enemy come from the plagues of classical antiquity. For example, the Spartans were accused of poisoning the springs that supplied water to Athens during the Peloponnesian war. One problem with these accounts is that it is often unclear what modern disease the various historical descriptions of 'plague' correspond to. Tainted water, though responsible for other infections, is unlikely to have been the source of the subsequent 'Plague of Athens' – it was more likely to have been caused by the crowding and congestion of the Athenian population behind the city walls during the siege. In the fourteenth century, the Tartars were said to have catapulted corpses of plague victims into the besieged city of Kaffa, causing outbreaks of plague within the city walls. However, if the 'plague' was what we now know as *Yersinia pestis,* the cause of bubonic plague, then the vectors would have been rats and lice, rather than infected corpses. However, neither the perpetrators nor the besieged would have understood that, and the resulting terror of contagion would nevertheless presumably have been great.

In fourteenth-century Europe, the 'Black Death' fanned existing anti-Semitism, and was widely believed to be the result of a Jewish conspiracy to deliberately poison the wells. Jews often traded in spices or as apothecaries, and many practiced as doctors, which raised additional suspicions and accusation of conspiracy. It is also possible that the belief that Jews were to blame for the Black Death was inspired or exacerbated by a visibly lower incidence of the plague among Jews, as they were segregated in their own urban quarters, cut off from the rodents on the wharves and the cattle in the countryside that were the main carriers of the disease. Jewish hygiene traditions and selective diets may well also have isolated them from the plague (Cantor, 2001). Similar reasons have been proposed as accounting for the Israelites escaping the Biblical plagues of Egypt.

The story of the decimation of the Native Americans through contact with Old World infections was recounted in Chapter 2. Without recourse to notions of divine intervention, both the indigenous South Americans and indeed the conquistadors themselves lacked any explanatory frameworks that could account for the huge numbers of deaths on one side while the other remained untouched. The infection of the South American indigenous populations was accidental, if not unwelcome from the conquistadors' point of view.

However, there is evidence from the eighteenth century that European settlers may have deliberately tried to infect Native Americans in North America by giving them blankets believed to be infected with smallpox. How often this primitive biological warfare was undertaken and with what rate of success is unclear. The extent to which Europeans understood how disease would be spread to the Native Americans is uncertain, and as in the South American case, it was more likely the accidental contact of two peoples with different patterns of immunity that wreaked such widespread damage (Kraut, 1994).

In the modern period, despite the appeal of biological weapons for terrorist groups, they have seldom been used by them. One exception occurred in 1981 when the followers of the Bhagwan Shree Rajneesh cult in The Dalles, Oregon, poisoned salad bars in restaurants with salmonella following a dispute over planning. 751 people were poisoned, making it the largest food poisoning outbreak in Oregon's history. The outbreak was at the time thought to be natural, and it was only a year later that ex-members of the cult accused their fellow members, leading to investigations that revealed the cult had experimented with various biological weapons agents at their commune, and which led to 20-year jail sentences for the perpetrators (Miller et al., 2001).

The Japanese Aum Shinrikiyo cult made another, more serious, attempt at bioterrorism by using sarin nerve agent to attack commuters on the Tokyo Subway in 1994 and 1995, killing 12 people and requiring more than 5,000 to be hospitalised. Their choice of *chemical* over *biological* terrorist weapons was apparently driven by the cult's failure to develop effective biological weapons. At its peak, the cult's worldwide membership was between 20,000 and 40,000 people, with an estimated net worth in March 1995 of about US$1.5 billion (Olson, 1999). The cult was adept at recruiting educated professionals – scientists and engineers – even though most were young and largely inexperienced. When police raided their facilities in 1995, they found enough sarin to kill an estimated 4.2 million people (Gardner, 2008). Members of the cult reportedly visited Zaire on the pretext of providing medical assistance to victims of the Ebola virus, with the actual objective of acquiring a sample to culture as a warfare agent (Stern, 1999). So despite the cult's explicitly stated objective of wanting to kill millions, and the cult's size, wealth, technical expertise and organisation, they found the technical hurdles of producing bioterrorism weapons prohibitively difficult.

So if bioterrorism had (so far) proved beyond the capability of even the most sophisticated terrorist groups, what then of their use or preparations for their use by governments? In 1969, President Nixon ended the US biological weapons programme, confining US research to defensive measures. In 1972, the USA, the Soviet Union and more than 100 other nations signed the Biological and Toxin Weapons Convention, prohibiting the development, production and stockpiling of deadly agents with no personal justification except for research into defensive measures such as vaccines, detectors and protective clothing (Miller et al., 2001). Yet in May 1992, President Yeltsin confirmed that the Soviet Union and later the Russian government had engaged in illegal development of biological agents through the nominally civilian secret biological weapons facilities of the 'Biopreparat' (Stern, 1999). One of these secret biological weapons facilities near the Soviet city of Sverdlovsk was the source of an accidental emission of a plume of aerosolised anthrax in April 1979, which led to the reported deaths of 64 people (Guillemin, 1999).

Saddam Hussein's Iraqi regime had admitted to developing an offensive biological weapons programme before the start of the first Gulf war, including bombs filled with botulinium toxin and anthrax spores, and prototype spray tanks capable of being mounted on remotely piloted aircraft (Danzig & Berkowsky, 1999). After its invasion of Kuwait in August 1990, Iraq engaged in what it called a 'crash programme' to produce large amounts of biological weapons (Stern, 1999).

In preparation for the first Gulf War, US troops were immunised against anthrax and botulinum and soldiers were issued with a five-day course of ciprofloxacin. Some 60,000 of the 697,000 US troops and 567 of the 45,000 UK troops who served in the first Gulf War subsequently complained that they developed so-called Gulf War Syndrome (also known as 'Saudi flu' or 'desert fever'). Iraq's admission that they had biological weapons added to the suspicions that Gulf War Syndrome was caused by either a toxic agent, or by the vaccines given, or a combination of both. Medical researchers investigated an infectious cause for the phenomenon, particularly as some family members of soldiers who had not been to the Gulf also reported symptoms, but the US Defense Department found no clear-cut evidence of transmission. Mainstream medical opinion believes that Gulf War Syndrome was the product of combat stress, which was physically and mentally acute in the Gulf war (Showalter, 1997).

After its defeat in February 1991, the Iraq government claimed to have destroyed its biological arsenal and research and production facilities that escaped destruction during the war were demolished by the United Nations Special Commission on Iraq (UNSCOM) in 1996 (Danzig & Berkowsky, 1999). Iraq was then subject to multiple intrusive inspections by UNSCOM. Yet '[e]ven with unrestricted access and a broad range of on-site measures, inspectors failed to uncover any unambiguous evidence of illicit biological weapons activity' (Kadlec et al., 1999: 96).

The pre-9/11 world

By the end of the first Gulf War in 1991, the US Congress had already passed two major statutes in an effort to control and prevent the use of biological weapons by domestic and international terrorists as well as by foreign nations: the Biological Weapons Act of 1989 and the Chemical and Biological Weapons Control and Warfare Elimination Act of 1991. Interest in the potential threat of bioweapons gradually increased in the decade between the first Gulf War and the 9/11 and anthrax attacks in 2001. There were fears of both the possible use of bioterrorism against US civilians, and of the possible use of bioweapons in battle by 'rogue states' such as Iraq. This ramping up of the risk discourse around bioweapons between 1991 and 2001 mirrors the increasing pitch of the contemporaneous discourse around EID, and as in the case of EID, prompted a range of legislation as well as a massive increase in US government spending on related research.

In February 1993, Muslim extremists detonated a car bomb in a car park below the North Tower of the World Trade Center in New York, killing six people and injuring over 1000. Then in April 1995, domestic terrorists linked to anti-government militias bombed a government building in Oklahoma City, killing 168 people and injuring over 800. In response to these attacks, and to the 1995 Aum Shinrikiyo attacks on the Tokyo subway, US counter-terrorism policy was updated in June 1995 as Presidential Decision Directive 39, which singled out as particularly worrying the use of nuclear, biological and chemical weapons (Stern, 1999). This was followed in 1996 by the US Anti-Terrorism Act, and in 1997 the US Congress established a comprehensive regulatory regime, regulated by the CDC, to control the domestic use of hazardous toxins and infectious agents (Ferguson, 1999).

In the same year, the Pentagon awarded a US$322 million ten-year contract for a plan to build up a stockpile of vaccines for smallpox, anthrax and other potential biological threats (Miller et al., 2001), and the then US Secretary of Defense, William S. Cohen, directed an increase in funding for counter-proliferation programmes by approximately US$1 billion over five years. Cohen decided to vaccinate all US forces personnel, active and reserve, against anthrax, a plan which would take over seven years to complete.

In August 1997, the *Journal of the American Medical Association* published a themed issue on biological weapons, which was co-edited by Joshua Lederberg, one of the original authors of the EID category. This special issue was later developed into a book, again edited by Lederberg, called *Biological Weapons: Limiting the Threat* (Lederberg, 1999). Lederberg had long been interested in the potential threat of biological weapons. During the Vietnam War, when he wrote a regular column in the *Washington Post*, he had called for curbs to germ warfare. In 1979, by then president of New York's Rockefeller University, he joined the Defense Science Board, a group of scientists who advised the US military. Lederberg had urged the first President Bush's administration to plan civil defences against a domestic germ attack in light of Saddam Hussein's threats, and some preparations were made as a result. In 1993, he had urged the Pentagon to broaden its biodefence agenda to include civilians, who he argued were vulnerable to attack, and in 1994 he briefed New York's Mayor Giuliani on the threat. Lederberg was also part of a secret federal programme known as *Reach Back*, a group of medical experts who wore bleepers so that they could be contacted in the event of a biological or chemical terrorist attack (Miller et al., 2001).

In the papers contained in both the 1997 special themed issue of the *Journal of the American Medical Association* and in the book that followed, there were two underlying premises. The first was that terrorist groups could manufacture bioterror weapons, if not easily, then at least feasibly. For example, one of the contributing authors to the *Biological Weapons* volume wrote:

> Unlike nuclear weapons, missiles or other advanced systems are not required for the delivery of biological weapons. Since aerosolisation is the predominant methods of dissemination, extraordinarily low-technology methods, including agricultural crop dusters, backpack sprayers, and even purse-size perfume atomizers will suffice. Small groups of people with modest finances and basic training in biology and engineering can develop an effective biological weapons capability. Recipes for making biological weapons are even available on the Internet. (Danzig & Berkowsky, 1999: 10)

Although this image of amateur enthusiasts apparently able to 'cook up' biological weapons agents *and* effective delivery methods is a powerful and frightening one, as discussed above, it was not borne out empirically by the Aum Shinrikiyo case.

The second premise of the discourse around bioterror by 1997 was that the likelihood of a bioterrorism attack was sufficiently great to warrant a very high level of concern, and by implication, that continued and increasing US government spending on bioweapons research and development was justified. Bioweapons research aimed to provide 'biodefence' measures, which would protect military forces should an attack occur in battle, for example protective suits and vaccinations for troops, such as Secretary of State Cohen's programme of anthrax vaccinations. However, it would have been impossible to provide protective suits and vaccinations for the entire US civilian population in the same way that was envisaged for protecting military personnel. Therefore, protecting civilians could only have been achieved by bolstering the existing civilian public health systems. This became known as 'biopreparedness': ensuring measures were in place that would aim to limit any damage should an attack occur, for example by ensuring that hospital emergency rooms, ambulance services and so on could cope following a civilian attack, rather than by protecting against such an attack in the first place (Rosenberg, 2002).

As described in Chapter 1, one of the key means by which the EID worldview became widely disseminated was through two popular science (non-fiction) books published in 1995, Laurie Garrett's *The Coming Plague* and Robert Preston's *The Hot Zone*. Both Garrett and Preston were given privileged access to many of the key figures who forged and promoted the EID category, in what was a (successful) attempt to put infectious diseases back on the scientific and cultural agenda. In fact, it was Lederberg who suggested to Preston the subject of the Ebola outbreak at Reston for *The Hot Zone* (Miller et al., 2001).

By 1997, as well as generating publications in the medical sphere, the subject of bioterrorism was also beginning to produce its own popular literature. Preston had learned of the US military's interest in a possible bioterrorist attack whilst writing *The Hot Zone,* and after its success, he turned his hand to fiction with *The Cobra Event* (Preston, 1997), a novel in which terrorists released advanced biological weapons to attack US civilians. Preston again used his contacts in the CDC, the FBI and elsewhere for his research for the novel. Lederberg is said to have advised Preston not only on technical detail – to revise his original story from anthrax weapons to a less plausible biologically engineered superbug (Miller et al., 2001) – but also on the story line – he advised him to let the assassin die of his virus at the end of the book, in order to deter possible real-life imitators (Sarasin, 2006). Similarly, Tom Clancy, in his 1996 novel *Executive Orders* (a sequel to his 1994 novel *Debt of Honor,* which presciently envisaged a hijacked 747 jet attacking the Capitol Building), imagined the president declaring a national state of emergency in response to a terrorist attack using an air-borne strain of Ebola virus (Annas, 2003).

President Clinton had read Tom Clancy's novels about bioterrorism and read *The Cobra Event* in early 1998. He discussed the impression Preston's novel had made on him with House Speaker Newt Gingrich and the Deputy Secretary of Defense, John Hamre. In April 1998, the President, together with his Defense Secretary, Attorney General, Health Secretary, CIA Director and National Security Advisor, held a meeting at the White House with seven leading US experts in biological weapons, including Lederberg. Clinton asked them what their assessment was of Preston's book. Several of the scientists later reported having stayed silent; one told the President that such an attack was possible. Lederberg told the President that any terrorist attack with an infectious agent would be 'a very serious event' and gave Clinton a copy of the August 1997 bioterrorism edition of the *Journal of the American Medical Association,* which he had edited (Miller et al., 2001).

Although those present at the meeting disagreed on the likelihood of a germ attack, all agreed that the USA had dangerously neglected its public health system, and argued that the alleged risk of bioterrorism presented a pressing need for extra resources in order that America would be prepared for a potential bioterror attack, as well as to deal with routine infectious diseases (Sarasin, 2006). As a result of the meeting, Clinton's rhetoric changed, and in 1999, at the National Academy of Sciences, with Lederberg at this side, Clinton announced his decision to ask congress for US$2.8 billion for biopreparedness, part of an overall request for US$10 billion for terrorism preparedness (Miller et al., 2001).

This meshing together of underlying concerns about the poor state of the US public health system and the imperative to protect against the threat of a (military) biological weapons or (civilian) bioterrorist attack continued when, in 1999, 950 public health officials, physicians and other medical personnel, together with government, military and intelligence experts, gathered for the first national *Symposium on Medical and Public Health Response to Bioterrorism.* The guiding force behind the symposium was D.A. Henderson, Dean of the School of Public Health at Johns Hopkins University and the founder and first director of the newly established Johns Hopkins Center for Civilian Biodefense Studies. (Henderson had been chief of the WHO Smallpox Eradication Unit in the 1960s.) The list of speakers again included Lederberg, and the presentations were later published in a July 1999 special issue of the CDC's own journal *Emerging Infectious Diseases* (Henderson, 1999). This meeting and the subsequent issue of *Emerging Infectious Diseases* included several lurid *what if* fictional papers hypothesising about possible smallpox attack scenarios and their aftermath on a fictional city called *Northeast*.

The level of biopreparedness for the widely anticipated bioterrorism attack against civilians was empirically tested with two 'desktop' operations. The first, called 'Operation Topoff', was carried out in May 2000 in Denver, Colorado and was the US administration's biggest ever disaster exercise, involving 20,000 high-ranking government officials. A simulated plague aerosol was said to have been covertly released, with over 2,000 cases of pneumonic plague and many deaths, and hundreds of secondary cases (Childress, 2003). The exercise ended in chaos and highlighted that in the face of either a natural or a malicious major infectious disease outbreak in a city like Denver, health services would quickly collapse (Sarasin, 2006).

The second biopreparedness exercise – called 'Dark Winter' – ran over two days in June 2001. It was organised by the Johns Hopkins Center for Civilian Biodefense Strategies, in collaboration with the Center for Strategic and International Studies, the Analytic Services Institute for Homeland Security, and the Oklahoma National Memorial Institute for the Prevention of Terrorism. Decision-makers were presented with a fictional scenario: that 3000 people were infected with the smallpox virus during simultaneous attacks on shopping malls in Oklahoma City, Philadelphia and Atlanta. They were then asked to react to the facts and context of the scenario, establish strategies and make policy decisions. As the event unfolded, they were told that in the worst-case scenarios, the fourth generation of cases could conceivably comprise as many as three million cases and as many as a million deaths. The scenario ended with the announcement that the *New York Times*, the *Washington Post* and *USA Today* had each received an anonymous letter demanding the removal of all US forces from Saudi Arabia and all warships from the Persian Gulf within one week. The letters threatened that failure to comply with the demands would result in new smallpox attacks on the US homeland as well as further attacks with anthrax and plague (O'Toole et al., 2002).

The plethora of scientific publications, books, meetings and 'biopreparedness' exercises that emerged throughout the 1990s would seem to indicate a consensus about the potential risk of a bioterror attack, but there was also a strand of expert opinion that thought the bioterror scenario unlikely. A 1988 book *Gene Wars: Military Control over the New*

Genetic Technologies (Piller & Yamamoto, 1988) had argued that germs could never be turned into viable weapons and that the threat was overstated. A later US Library of Congress report on the subject, in 1999, had similarly concluded that '[w]eapons of mass destruction are significantly harder to produce or obtain than what is commonly depicted in the press and today they probably remain beyond the reach of most terrorist groups' (Gardner, 2008: 304).

In May 2001, the *American Journal of Public Health* published a series of articles on the threat of, and response to, a potential bioterror attack. By this time, proposals to protect against such a threat were provoking sharp debate (Gieger, 2001). As in the earlier *Emerging Infectious Diseases* (journal) special on the subject, papers included *what if?* hypotheses about fictional terrorist attack scenarios involving anthrax and causing 32,000 deaths (Wetter et al., 2001). One connected theme that ran through these papers, and through Lederberg's book, was the chronic and worsening neglect of the US public health infrastructure, and the 'dual use' of biopreparedness: 'Physicians and local health services... are in the front lines to deal with health emergencies. This same apparatus is needed to deal with natural disease outbreaks' (Lederberg, 1999: 7). Thus some commentators argued that biopreparedness programmes would provide a badly needed resources bonanza for public health, with increases in funding and personnel that would make it easier to deal with unintentional food-borne and chemical incidents, as well as with EID (Henretig, 2001). However, on the other side of the debate, were those who argued that the probability of biological or chemical attack was very close to zero, and spending vast sums of public money on biopreparedness and the 'militarisation' of US public health could hamper efforts to prevent disease among those most poorly served by the US medical system (Sidel et al., 2001).

While there was an ongoing debate within public health circles about the wisdom of diverting attention from the poor state of the US public health system towards biopreparedness just before the 9/11 attacks, within US government circles the argument seems to have been won. In early 2001, Congress authorised the spending of over US$500 million for bioterrorism preparedness through the Public Health Threats and Emergencies Act (Hodge & Gostin, 2003). The received wisdom of the 'inevitability' of a bioterror attack against the USA trickled down from the biomedical journals and US government agencies into the mass media, aided by articles such as Laurie Garrett's *The Nightmare of Bioterrorism*, published in January 2001 in *Foreign Affairs* (Garrett, 2001).

On 5 September 2001, a letter from Lederberg was read to a meeting of the US Senate Committee on Foreign Relations, in which he wrote:

Considerable harm could be done (on the scale of, say, a thousand casualties) by rank amateurs. Terrorist groups, privately or state-sponsored, with funds up to US$1 million, could mount massive attacks of ten or 100 times that scale. Important to keep in mind: if the ultimate casualty roster is 1,000, there will have been 100,000 or 1,000,000 at risk in the target zone, legitimately demanding prophylactic attention, and in turn a draconian triage. (Childress, 2003: 76)

In the same week, the US government confirmed press reports that the Defense Intelligence Agency was preparing to develop a new and more virulent strain of anthrax thought to be in the possession of Russia, with the aim of preventing a successful attack by discovering the potential of actual offensive devices. At the same time, the CIA was reported to have built a replica of a biological weapons dispersal device developed by the Soviet Union, again for defensive study purposes (Moreno, 2003). By early September 2001, it was taken as 'common sense' that US civilians faced a clear, present and inevitable danger from terrorists using anthrax, smallpox and other biological weapons.

After the attacks

Given the pitch of the risk discourse about the threat of a bioterrorist attack in the years and months leading up to September 2001, it is perhaps not surprising that the US authorities' attention was initially focused elsewhere when a more low-tech, but equally stunning attack occurred. Just minutes after planes crashed into The World Trade Center, the National Guard was mobilised to test the air for biological or chemical agents (Sarasin, 2006). None were found, but within a week the anthrax letters had been posted and a new era had dawned, one in which the long anticipated but largely hypothetical threat of bioterrorism had become a 'reality'.

One of the consequences of the anthrax attacks was a move to introduce new legislation which would put sweeping powers in the hands of public health officials in the event of a public health emergency such as bioterrorism attacks, as well in the event of an epidemic of an EID. At the request of the CDC, on 30 October 2001, a Model State Emergency Health Powers Act was drafted by lawyers and academics at

The Center for Law and the Public's Health at Georgetown and Johns Hopkins Universities in collaboration with members of national organisations representing governors, legislators, attorneys general and health commissioners. The Model Act's foundations in part lay in the lessons derived from the theoretical exercises such as 'Dark Winter' (Gostin et al., 2002) and it was intended to be adapted for use by individual states.

The act bore the marks of having official backing of the CDC, and, unsurprisingly, the press saw it as a government initiative (Bayer & Colgrove, 2003). The Model Act took on a life of its own, and it required considerable work on the part of members of patient advocacy groups to explain why such draconian provisions would be unnecessary and counterproductive (Annas, 2003), and would infringe in times of emergency what in normal circumstances would be taken as basic liberty rights (May, 2005). Nevertheless, by June 2002, legislative bills based on the Model Act had been introduced in 34 states and the District of Columbia, and 16 states and the District of Columbia had enacted a version of the act (Gostin et al., 2002).

Another consequence of the anthrax attacks was a huge rise in US government funding for biopreparedness measures. The CDC announced that it was to distribute US\$1 billion to individual states, allocated on the basis of evidence of efforts made to provide the legal infrastructure and to prepare systematic response plans for bioterrorism prevention (Hodge & Gostin, 2003).

At the *Interscience Conference on Antimicrobial Agents and Chemotherapy* in San Diego in September 2002, Anthony Fauci, the Director of the US National Institute for Allergies and Infectious Diseases (NIAID), told participants that in 2000–1 the National Institute of Health (NIH) spent between US\$50 and US\$75 million on biodefence, but for 2003 the government had earmarked US\$1.74 billion, amounting to the largest single increase of any discipline, disease or institute in the history of the NIH (Ashraf, 2002).

One of these biopreparedness measures was the National Smallpox Vaccination Program, announced by President Bush in December 2002, ironically in the very year that the World Health Assembly had earmarked for the destruction of the remaining stocks of the variola virus (Henderson & Fenner, 2001). The programme's aim was extraordinary: to vaccinate a million people against smallpox, a disease that no longer existed, with a vaccine that posed some well-known risks. The vaccination was to be offered to some categories of civilians and administered to members of the military and US government representatives in high risk areas of the world. However, February 2003, the footprints of the original plan had been removed from federal websites, leaving only the bare bones of a recommendation for immunisation of 'smallpox response teams' (Alcabes, 2009). In June 2003, the Advisory Committee on Immunization Practices recommended bringing pre-event smallpox vaccination to a close.

A 2005 IOM report into the smallpox vaccination programme criticised the communication from the usually open and transparent CDC as 'constrained by unknown external influences'. As the programme ran into difficulties, and appeared to fall short of initial expectations, goals were not clarified or revised in any substantive way. There was no assessment of the programme's outcomes in terms of actual smallpox preparedness achieved, no review of lessons learned, no accounting of what had been done with the opportunities for scientific research (Committee on Smallpox Vaccination Program Implementation, 2005).

The same IOM report pointed out that the smallpox vaccination programme was created just as the administration was beginning to build a case for war against Iraq. The report suggested that a rationale for the programme can be inferred from statements by President Bush, for example, when he said in December 2002, 'we believe that regimes hostile to the USA may possess this dangerous virus'. Other unnamed officials subsequently revealed that the regime in question was Iraq. Another factor that cemented the perceived link between the war and stoking fears of smallpox was that efforts to implement the vaccination programme essentially came to a halt once President Bush declared 'the end of major combat operations in Iraq' in April 2003. By July 2003, only 38,004 civilians had been vaccinated, far below the president's stated goal of 500,000, and in August only five new individuals were vaccinated. Afterwards, the programme languished, and the federal government became silent on its status and future (Wynia, 2006).

Another biopreparedness measure was 'Project Bioshield', proposed by President Bush in his State of the Union speech in January 2003. This was a permanent fund of over US$6 billion to develop and produce vaccines for Ebola, plague and other potential bioterror agents. In order to incentivise pharmaceutical companies, the president promised a market for the resulting products of their research, even if they were never used. In response, the pharmaceutical industry demanded higher guaranteed profits, and protection from liability in case of adverse side-effects (King, 2003b). The Project Bioshield Act was passed by the US Congress in 2004.

In 2003, the new biosecurity discourse came of age when its own journal was launched: *Biosecurity and Bioterrorism: Biodefense Strategy, Practice and Science*, with the aim being to foster 'a deeper understanding of the threat posed by biological weapons and to broaden the spectrum of people who are knowledgeable in these realms' (O'Toole & Inglesby, 2003: 2). Within the so-called 'war on terror', spending on biopreparedness, with US$5.2 billion spent in 2004 alone, came second only to direct military funding. Biopreparedness was prioritised over other US domestic political issues and concern about bioterrorism transformed public health, neglected for decades, into a central component of national security (May 2005).

Apart from the domestic US resource allocation issues that were raised by biopreparedness, the graver consequence of the anthrax attacks was that they provided the justification for the war against Iraq in 2003. With the anthrax letters coming so soon after the 9/11 attacks, it was perhaps inevitable that the issue of bioterrorism would be elided with 9/11, although the anthrax letters were an entirely separate and extraordinary phenomenon. It was clear to the US authorities within weeks after the anthrax attacks had occurred that the source was more likely a domestic terrorist, despite the (perhaps deliberately) clumsy attempt by the perpetrator(s) to implicate Islamist extremists. It has been pointed out, for example, that any native Arabic speaker would translate *Allah akbar* as 'God is great', not 'Allah is great'. The Internet buzzed with conspiracy theories, proposing that the anthrax letters were a US government-backed plot to link the 9/11 attacks to Saddam Hussein.

There is no doubt that the Bush administration had been, at the very least, considering war with Iraq before 9/11. It is also reasonable to assume that the anthrax attacks were planned for many months before 9/11, for who could produce weapons-grade anthrax in a week? However, the idea of the involvement of the US government in the anthrax attacks seems as far-fetched as other 9/11 conspiracy theories doing the rounds of the Internet at the time: such as 'the Jews' were behind the attacks. Less far-fetched is the notion that the hawks in the US administration, with the aid of British Prime Minister Tony Blair, used the anthrax attacks to build a conceptual bridge, one that could not otherwise have been built, between the religious fanatics responsible for 9/11 and the secular dictatorship in Iraq, thus 'proving' the 'reality' of the threat to the 'world' from Saddam Hussein's Weapons of Mass Destruction (Sarasin, 2006).

On 5 February 2003, in a pivotal speech arguing for war against Iraq, Colin Powell showed the UN Security Council delegates a small container of white powder. He said:

Less than a teaspoon of dry anthrax, a little bit about this amount – this is just about the amount of a teaspoon – less than a teaspoonful of dry anthrax in an envelope shutdown the United States Senate in the fall of 2001. This forced several hundred people to undergo emergency medical treatment and killed two postal workers just from an amount just about this quantity that was inside of an envelope.

Partly as a result of Powell's speech, the second war against Iraq – 'Operation Iraqi Freedom' – went ahead on 19 March. After the war, UNSCOM failed to find Weapons of Mass Destruction in Iraq. Powell is reported to have later regretted his speech at the UN, which he regarded as a 'permanent blot' on his record (Weisman, 2005).

The bioterrorism myth

There was thus increased interest in bioterrorism long before the 2001 anthrax letter attacks. What conclusions can we draw from this interest about the way the discourse around infectious diseases has changed in the early twenty-first century? The first conclusion is that the issue of bioterror illustrates how the EID worldview had become established to the extent that it became the 'natural' frame of reference to conceptualise the threat of bioterrorism. On a denotative level, many of the issues seem the same or similar whether faced with the threat of an emerging infectious disease or with bioterrorism.

As discussed in Chapter 4, when epidemics of infectious diseases threaten 'us', *others* (migrants, foreigners, or other already stigmatised groups within the host society) are usually held responsible. 'They' may be already living amongst 'us', or are at least only a plane journey away. This blaming discourse, based on the antimony of the healthy self and the diseased *other*, is transposed onto the bioterrorism discourse, as are the militarised metaphors used to describe infectious disease, echoing the way that military and espionage metaphors are used to describe the immune system – infections, invasions, terrorist 'cells', detection, defence, eradication and so on. The potential bioterrorist, like the infected *other*, threatens both individual citizens and the body politic from within or without. The response in both cases is to limit migration and to increase border security, and to introduce draconian legislation to limit civil freedoms in the name of public health and internal security. In other words, the twenty-first century response to the threat both of the infected *other* and of the bioterrorist is to revert to a more primitive group instinct: to regard outsiders with suspicion and fear and to seek to exclude them.

The *National Security Strategy of the USA* of September 2002 argued that strengthening the emergency management systems of the USA would make the country better able to manage not only terrorism, but also all infectious disease outbreaks and mass casualty dangers. The border control would stop not only terrorists but improve efficient movement of legitimate traffic. The issues of conventional terrorism, bioterrorism, EID and immigration were thus all elided. Illegal immigrants and the threat from EID they were felt to pose were placed *on the same level* as the threat posed by terrorists and bioterrorism (Sarasin, 2006).

Fears of terrorism prompted the US Congress to pass measures tightening control of the borders and intensifying the scrutiny and surveillance of immigrants (Fairchild, 2004). Similar measures were instituted in many European countries and elsewhere. This 'securitisation' of the discourse around migration has its foundations in fear of infection, and echoes the threat of the Jewish *other* poisoning the wells in the time of the Black Death. It is cemented by the fear that immigrants may be supporters of insurgencies or potential contributors to uprisings and terrorist activities, and has led to 'ethnic profiling' and subsequent deportation. That migrants are a security risk has come to be understood as fact, and no attempt is made to debate the notion in the media (Ibrahim, 2005).

As well as a transposition of blaming discourse and measures to exclude immigrants, another strand of the bioterrorism discourse connects with that around EID: that of the risk posed by (the bioterrorists') misuse of technology. The bioterrorist

> seizes 'our' biotechnology – a symbol of American modernity and economic might – and transforms it into a political weapon. He personifies American loss of control over not only its national borders, but also its scientific achievements. On a deeper level he challenges the moral neutrality of those achievements, exposing what has come to be called the 'dual use' dilemma: greater understanding and control over infectious diseases inevitably leads to greater opportunity for transforming those diseases into weapons. (King, 2003b: 438)

The interest in bioterrorism increased as the interest in EID such as AIDS declined through the 1990s. Yet another, perhaps paradoxical, conclusion can also be drawn from the interest in bioterrorism in the 1990s and early twenty-first century: namely that the EID worldview had become so embedded as to become 'common sense', even banal. In coining the EID category in the early 1990s, one of the central motives was to gain popular and political attention, and thus funding, for esoteric issues such as the rise of antibiotic-resistant bacterial infections in hospitals or the re-emergence of tuberculosis amongst the indigent poor in American cities. Attention for these issues was garnered by 'sexing up' the issue. The new classification of infectious diseases as EID aggregated issues like antibiotic resistance with the newsworthiness of entirely separate phenomenon like HIV/AIDS and 'far-flung' exotic diseases such as Ebola. This strategy worked extraordinarily well and succeeded in attracting the attention of the news media, the public, politicians and biomedical research funding bodies.

The thinking and strategy behind the EID success was then extended to bioterror and biopreparedness. As with the construction of the EID category, one of the main drivers for those involved in promoting the threat of bioterrorism was the perceived secondary benefit of badly needed finances directed to the US public health system. Increased funding for biopreparedness was said to have a 'dual use', insofar as the chief method of ensuring that civilian populations could be protected in the event of an attack was to ensure that there was sufficient capacity in emergency rooms, ambulance services and so on. Thus biopreparedness initiatives were said to lend strength to public health infrastructure and its ability to address EID.

However, although biopreparedness initiatives may have provided many a research scientist and their laboratories with new seams of financial resources to mine, the hope that biopreparedness would lead to gains for the US public health system, or indeed for global public health, now seem naive. Many argued that the infrastructure needed for biopreparedness was the same as that required to protect against EID. However, the focus of biopreparedness was on research into, and stockpiling of, treatments and vaccines: the billions of dollars spent on Project Bioshield, for example, and the provision of enough smallpox vaccine for every US citizen.

Meanwhile, the number of US hospital emergency departments was declining, because they were being closed due to the financial drain they represented to hospitals, as those tens of millions of Americans without health insurance present there as a last resort when they lack any other access to primary health care. This dire situation was only likely to be exacerbated by the significant outlay on equipment, facilities and supplies for biopreparedness that may never be used, with little prospect of financial compensation for these expenditures (May, 2005). Despite initial hopes, actual bioterror defence spending was not targeted at improving the US public health infrastructure, and the disproportionate level of US government support for high-cost domestic biopreparedness led to inevitable comparisons with the lack of conviction surrounding federal support for reforms such as inclusive health coverage (Eckenwiler, 2003). Countries other than the USA – for example, in Europe – took some basic precautions against bioterrorism, such as stockpiling smallpox vaccine, but there was nowhere near the funding avalanche of the USA (Enserink & Kaiser, 2005).

In the climate immediately following the terrorist attacks, attention was increasingly focused away from EID and onto the threat from terrorism, both bioterrorism and its more 'conventional' form. For example, at the 2002 *Interscience Conference on Antimicrobial Agents and Chemotherapy,* the dominant theme was the US medical community's response to bioterrorism, a concern for public health by then regarded as equally as pressing and crucial as the previous central public health concern, HIV/AIDS (Ashraf, 2002). Thus the 'emerging or re-emerging' category was extended to include a third element: *deliberately emerging diseases,* now incorporating those infectious diseases intentionally introduced as agents of bioterror, such as anthrax. For the scientific and public health audiences, the three categories – *emerging, re-emerging or deliberately emerging diseases* – came to be treated in much the same way (Fauci, 2006).

In terms of post-Cold War era medical research programmes, the bonanza of US government funding thrown at biopreparedness came second only to cancer. As a result, scientists in the field of infectious diseases altered their research priorities in order to tap into the huge pot of money. Most of the applied research supported by the government on drugs and vaccines for potential bioterrorism agents would have had little effect on the diseases that pose the gravest threat to people. The 'spin offs' promised by Anthony Fauci, Director of the NIAID were negligible or non-existent. Vaccine research is almost always pathogen specific, as are most drugs used to combat viral diseases, and the number of people worldwide who suffer from smallpox, botulism, Ebola or anthrax 'wouldn't fill up the TB ward in a small African city' (Goozner, 2003). Far from pursuing spin off, many scientists simply shifted their priorities to follow the money. There were also concerns expressed that the number of laboratories and people working on potential bioterror agents would actually increase the risk of a bioterrorism attack by a disgruntled scientist (Enserink & Kaiser, 2005).

In 2005, there was a mutiny by over 700 researchers who had served on NIH review groups or received grants reviewed by those groups. They signed an open letter in the journal *Science* to Elias Zerhouni, director of the NIH in which they complained that microbial research with any significance for public health was threatened by the prioritisation of NIAID of biodefence – grants that referenced tularaemia, anthrax, plague, glanders, meliodosis and brucellosis had increased by 1,500 per cent between 1996 and 2001. They also argued that while institutions and investigators that had followed this money, between 1996 and 2005 the number of grants for non-biodefence microbial research had decreased by 41 per cent, and grants for research into pathogenic organisms had decreased by 27 per cent (Altman et al., 2005).

Bioterrorism provides a stunning exemplar of how much infectious disease had become politicised at the end of the twentieth century. The threat of bioterrorism was cultivated into mythic status for over ten years. When the anthrax letter attacks 'proved' that the threat was 'real', the hawks in the US government then used the myth of bioterrorism to justify the war against Iraq. But many scientists and public health officials also colluded in the fantasy, hoping that spending on biopreparedness would prove 'dual use' and serve their aims, namely to redirect funding to woefully neglected public health. Eventually it became clear that bioterrorism was diverting money and talent away from public health, rather than directing resources towards it. The following, final chapter will discuss how public health came to be seen as a security issue, and will contextualise the risk that infectious diseases pose, not to the security of the USA and developed world states, but to the poor in the developing world.

8
EID, Security and Global Poverty

The EID category was coined as an attempt to refocus the scientific community, US politicians and the public, onto the threat that infectious diseases continued to pose (to Americans). The authors of this new category were astonishingly successful in achieving their goal. The term 'emerging infectious diseases' may remain obscure for most lay people, yet even so, the central concept behind the EID concept has gained wide currency in both scientific and lay discourse. That central idea is that infectious diseases are no longer a thing of the past, but are re-emerging to threaten 'us' (in the developed world). The proposition that infectious diseases are re-emerging has become, in effect, common sense.

As discussed in the previous chapter, since it was coined in the early 1990s, the EID concept has also become the template by which new concerns about bioterrorism came to be understood. However, as well as concerns about the possibility of terrorists deliberately using infectious germs as weapons, by the beginning of the twenty-first century, even naturally occurring epidemics of EID were also being described as a security threat.

EID as a security threat

During the Cold War, the term 'security' was understood in the sense of 'national security', as the absence of armed conflict, and 'security' was polarised around the ideological interests of the two superpowers. However, through the 1990s, the USA, together with international bodies such as the UN, began to give more attention to threats arising from mass migration, civil unrest and localised wars. 'Security' became increasingly redefined in terms of 'human security' (Chen & Narasimhan, 2003; Heymann, 2003). Issues that degraded the quality of life, such as demographic pressures or lack of access to resources, were thus recast as 'security threats'. This broadening of the notion of security was also extended to EID because of their disruptive potential. A number of think-tank reports linked EID directly with US national interests. For example, the Santa Monica-based RAND Corporation, which argued that threats to US security arose not only from military aggression, but increasingly from non-traditional, transnational so-called 'grey area' phenomenon, such as the drug trade, terrorism, and infectious diseases (Brower & Chalk, 2003).

In 2000, a US National Intelligence Council report, *The Global Infectious Disease Threat and its Implications for the United States*, argued:

> New and re-emerging infectious diseases will pose a rising global health threat and will complicate US and global security over the next 20 years. These diseases will endanger US citizens at home and abroad, threaten US armed forces deployed overseas, and exacerbate social and political instability in key countries and regions in which the United States has significant interests. (National Intelligence Council, 2000: 5)

Although all EID were said to pose a threat to peace and security in the US and the rest of the world, it was HIV/AIDS specifically that was regarded as a particular threat to security. In 2000, the United Nations Security Council passed a resolution addressing HIV/AIDS as a threat to international peace and security, to the viability of states and to economic development. This was the first time that the council had portrayed a health issue as a threat to security. Their concerns were focused on certain countries in Africa, and increasingly on Ukraine, China and India. In the same year, President Clinton provoked much controversy and comment when he announced that HIV/AIDS constituted a threat to US national security interests.

HIV/AIDS evidently poses a threat to the security of certain countries in sub-Saharan Africa, in terms of the pandemic's potential to damage their political institutions, military capacity, police force and health-care systems. The pandemic also has the potential to unravel traditional systems of social support in developing countries, and undermine development gains as skilled workers are lost and foreign investment reduced (Heymann, 2003). The argument is made that HIV/AIDS, combined with poverty, can cause states to fail, and failed states are unable to stem the growth of terrorist groups such as Al Qaeda within their borders, which in turn threaten the security of the USA. However, there are still several leaps of unsubstantiated argument involved in connecting the HIV/AIDS epidemic *in Africa* to a putative threat posed to the security of Americans *in America*. Indeed, subsequent analyses have also rejected the notion that the disease was likely to cause widespread social instability in other countries, for example in Russia, where the disease is largely confined to certain groups (Ingram, 2005).

This 'securitisation' of EID poses several difficulties: One danger is that portraying EID as a 'security threat' works against ongoing efforts to normalise attitudes to those people affected by them, such as people living with HIV/AIDS. Another danger of framing EID in the language of security is that it risks pushing responses to them away from civil society, such as humanitarian relief for the poor, and towards immigration, military and intelligence services, with their power to override civil liberties. The discourse around HIV/AIDS and security in Africa often focuses on the role of the African armed forces, which are regarded as a 'high-risk' group. This has led to international policy interventions to educate soldiers and raise awareness of 'safer sex', when the most obvious behaviour change that needs to take place is for soldiers to stop raping women (Elbe, 2008).

In 2003, following the designation of HIV/AIDS as a threat to global security, and also as a result of lobbying by evangelical Christians and African-American groups with long-standing interests in HIV/AIDS and Africa, President Bush launched the President's Emergency Plan for AIDS Relief (PEPFAR). Bush pledged US$15 billion over five years, US$1 billion of which was earmarked for the Global Fund to Fight HIV/AIDS, Tuberculosis and Malaria. The money was to be channelled through the US State Department and US embassies rather than through established international health agencies (Ingram, 2007). As a result of PEPFAR, 970,000 people were able to access anti-retroviral drugs, compared to 5,000–10,000 previously. PEPFAR aimed to prevent seven million HIV infections, to provide treatment for two million people, and care for ten million AIDS patients (Fauci, 2006). Before the 2007 G8 summit, Bush announced a further US$30 billion to continue the programme. In July 2008 the US Congress increased the PEPFAR budget by a further US$39 billion for AIDS, as well as US$5 billion for malaria and US$4 billion for tuberculosis (Kaufmann, 2009).

However, PEPFAR has been heavily criticised for the way its funding was directed towards initiatives judged on moral rather than scientific criteria. For instance, PEPFAR insisted that every recipient of aid money sign a declaration expressly promising not to have any involvement with sex workers (Goldacre, 2008); 50 per cent of the money was channelled through non-governmental organisations (NGOs) and faith-based organisations; and 33 per cent of prevention funds (US$1.06 billion) was earmarked for programmes promoting abstinence from sex until marriage. PEPFAR's moralising was directed at African societies who were themselves undergoing religious revivals on the model of the American evangelical mega-churches. For many, PEPFAR was a cynical attempt at 'soft hegemony' by the Bush administration. Although the entire project was funded by the US taxpayer, it was called the 'President's' plan, rather than the US (taxpayer's) plan, or the global plan for AIDS relief. PEPFAR was announced while the USA was preparing for war in Iraq, in an atmosphere of international protests against US militarism and accusations of xenophobia. Bush called PEPFAR 'a work of mercy – to help the people of Africa', and it was designed to rebut these accusations (Pisani, 2008).

The resistance to initiatives such as PEPFAR as 'imperialist' was also expressed in relation to the WHO-sponsored campaign to eradicate poliomyelitis. The campaign, launched in 1988, had led to a worldwide decline in annual polio cases from 35,251 to 1499 by 2005. At one stage the WHO was predicting that polio would be eradicated by 2005, although cases of wild polio virus continued to be reported from Northern Nigeria. The campaign then had to be suspended in Niger and Nigeria in 2005 as a result of local resistance, and soon polio outbreaks began to occur again there, and spread to other African countries and subsequently to Asia. Although resistance to the polio vaccine has been widely attributed to Nigerian Muslims' beliefs that the vaccine was contaminated with anti-fertility substances as a plot to reduce Muslim populations, there were also other more complex reasons for their refusals to vaccinate. Local people questioned the focus on polio, the vaccine for which was free, which they felt diverted resources from other more pressing primary health care needs, such as malaria, the medicines for which they had to pay for. Local resistance to polio vaccination was based partly on the feeling that malaria and measles were a more serious threat to their children, and people felt they had no say in which health problems were being addressed (Renne, 2006).

EID and post-colonialism

The 'securitisation' of infectious diseases, and the moralising of PEPFAR, echoed the colonial and missionary projects of the nineteenth century. Historical parallels can be drawn between EID and the creation of another medical speciality – Tropical Medicine – a hundred years earlier. While white Europeans could settle the Americas, South Africa, New Zealand and Australia, their inability to deal with malaria and other tropical diseases meant that they were unable to displace native populations in Africa, where Europeans had to limit themselves to the role of financiers and supervisors. Central Africa remained a black continent only because it was the white man's grave (Dubos, 1959). The founding of Schools of Tropical Medicine in Liverpool in 1898 and in London in the following year were thus explicitly linked to colonial politics and imperial expansionism. The Victorian debate about Tropical Medicine centred on the capacity of white bodies to adjust to the pathogenic, medical, moral and cultural climate of the tropical world. The tropics was a place where temperance and morality, such as avoiding inter-racial liaisons, were regarded as essential for survival as acquired immunity and medication (Livingstone, 1999).

Ignorance of actual distribution of disease in colonial populations led nineteenth-century medical and social theorists to assume that the different races were immune to diseases of their homelands, and equally that races would be susceptible to foreign diseases (Anderson, 1996). Although the export of Western medicine (and religion) was one of the chief justifications offered for colonialism as a humanitarian endeavour (King, 2002), in fact the European powers', and later US, interests in colonial public health were to assure the health of white soldiers, traders and settlers. Only later was the focus widened to include the health of indigenous populations, although except for male workers, these improvements were a negligible and secondary side-effect.

If the late nineteenth-century creation of Tropical Medicine related to the vulnerability of white populations to tropical infections in colonial outposts, another concern for the Victorians was that the poor on their own doorsteps also posed a risk of contagion. Again and again, Dickens's novels contain warnings of how all strata of society were vulnerable to the diseases that rampaged, unchecked, through the indigenous poor. For example, the central character of *Bleak House*, Esther Summerson, who, in a chance encounter, contracts smallpox from a street sweeper. While the Victorians dreaded smallpox and TB, their greatest fear of contagion from the poor related to cholera. One of the most shocking revelations about the London cholera epidemic of 1855 was that it happened in the rich district of St James, while the nearby abjectly poor district of St Giles was practically untouched. Londoners thought that if people in fashionable St James could die of cholera, it could happen anywhere (Gilbert, 2005). 'Asiatic' cholera exposed the fault lines of the newly industrialised society. Victorians conceptualised it as an exotic

Indian disease that flourished in the similar conditions found in English cities. A characteristic side-effect of cholera was that its victims' skin became dry and dark, like an African. In a form of reverse colonisation, cholera thus transformed the English into a race of 'savages' (O'Conner, 2000).

Over a century later, we find that the EID worldview is similarly obsessed with the notion that origin of infection resides in other nations or in marginalised groups at home, and seeks to prevent 'leakage' from infected *others* into 'the general population'. This notion holds as much for gay or bisexual men with HIV as it does for asylum seekers with TB, for Africans with Ebola or for Chinese with SARS. But just as the 'War on Drugs' was always more of a war on drug users, so the battle to exclude EID becomes less of a battle to combat these diseases *in situ* (by improving the health of the poor and marginalised in developing nations and at home), and becomes more of a battle to stigmatise and exclude the *other*.

Developed world EID

In Chapter 1 there was a description of the different factors that were said to be behind the emergence or re-emergence of infectious diseases. But by aggregating such a wide range of different diseases and their different causes, the EID worldview obscures the enormous differences in the way that these diseases affect rich and poor, both in developed and developed countries.

Some of the factors causing the emergence of new infectious diseases are more pertinent to or exclusively affect people in the developed world. For example, the demographic change in Western countries towards an ageing population has led to a growing number of immuno-compromised people vulnerable to infections. In the developed world, changes in the susceptibility of older people account for most of the apparent increases in infectious diseases. For example, the 58 per cent increase in deaths from infectious diseases in the USA between 1980 and 1992 was largely due to an increased infectious disease mortality rate among people over 65 from respiratory infections. The exception is people with AIDS, who account for most of the infections in those between 24 and 44 (Schwartz & Yogev, 1996). The peak of incidence of new infectious diseases reported in the 1980s in the USA and other developed countries are thus AIDS-related opportunistic infections (Jones et al., 2008).

One of the factors said to cause diseases to emerge is use of technology, particularly in medicine and in food production. Again this is more of an issue in developed countries: Some nosocomial infections, such as MRSA, are more common in those developed countries where there is a greater use of medical technology such as intravenous catheters, and antibiotics which are then used to treat infections associated with these technologies. Some food-borne pathogens, such as BSE/vCJD, are also confined largely to the developed world. Although concerns about travel importing EID tends to be framed in terms of poor migrants transporting infections from developing countries to developed ones, rich travellers to developing world countries are also likely to carry certain infections home with them. Half of all tourists and business travellers from industrialised countries who travel to developing countries fall ill with diarrhoea, 50 per cent of those cases are caused by *E. Coli*, 20 per cent by viruses, particularly noroviruses and ten per cent are due to protozoa such as *Giardia*, with the remainder due to other bacteria such as salmonella and shigellae (Kaufmann, 2009).

The rise in reports of infectious diseases in developed countries is also in part an artefact of improved diagnostic and laboratory techniques. For example, the original IOM report includes one of the 'emerging' infections as the bacterium *Helicobacter pylori,* which, in the 1980s, was discovered to be the cause of most gastric ulcers. Yet there is no evidence that the frequency of *H. pylori* had increased. Similarly, there has been an increase in reports of diarrhoea caused by the food-borne pathogen *Cyclosporidium,* but this increase in incidence relates to improved laboratory techniques which, from the mid-1980s, allowed for more accurate diagnoses.

A further factor likely to cause the emergence of infectious diseases in developed countries is microbial adaptation and change. Antigenic shifts, such as occur with the influenza virus, can lead to more virulent strains to which people are naive, and the virus thus spreads until either natural or vaccine-induced immunity increases. This might explain the recent variations of invasive group A streptococcal infections ('flesh-eating bacteria') and the emergence of toxic shock syndrome (Schwartz & Yogev, 1996). Other infections that fall under the category of 'emerging' are as old as human civilisation but have changed in some way, such as TB. But usually when microbes have evolved, it is because humans have played a large role in enhancing their pathogenicity through ecological or demographic changes (Morse, 1995).

International travel and commerce are often blamed as a cause of cases of 'exotic' diseases such as Hantaan viruses to emerge in the USA. While some EID, such as SARS, were spread by international travel, the ability of an infection to become established and spread once introduced to a new area still depends on other factors being favourable to it. For example, in August 1987, there was an outbreak of group A meningococcal meningitis during the annual hajj pilgrimage to Mecca, Saudi Arabia, which resulted in an attack rate among American pilgrims of 640 per 100,000. Yet there was no subsequent epidemic in the USA (Moore et al., 1988). Similarly, sporadic cases of malaria have been reported in Europeans with no history of travel to malarial countries but who lived near to airports, and mosquitoes travelling in the wheel bays of international airplane flights have been suggested as the cause. However, these mosquito vectors cannot thrive and reproduce in colder climates, so the conditions for the disease to spread further are not present. Similarly, developed world levels of sanitation would prevent a faecal–oral disease such as cholera spreading to epidemic levels.

Another factor said to lead to the emergence of epidemics of infectious disease is infections transported in the bodies of infected plane travellers who may not yet display symptoms. The so-called *stepping off a plane* scenario was a feature of the early Ebola reporting and has been a recurring *motif* in the reporting of other EID. There have been well-documented cases of a single plane journey transporting a disease from one country to another, for example with SARS. However, as Paul Farmer points out, 'transmission of this sort, though dramatic and well-documented, is rare. Far more common is the... hidden-away suffering of a family that will never board a plane to any destination' (Farmer, 2005: 127). The point is that most people affected by EID are unlikely to *step onto a plane* in the first place because most EID primarily affect the poor. Yet the dread of the poor, of immigrants or of 'foreigners', as a source of infection (of the rich) persists as an enduring theme in the history of infectious diseases. The *stepping off a plane scenario* is one modern incarnation of this fear of contagion.

The definition of EID usually rests on increased incidence (the number of newly diagnosed cases during a specific time period) rather than on prevalence (the number of cases alive in a population on a certain date). Investigators have often presented cases encountered in their practice and suggested an increased frequency of a disease, but such extrapolations may not be valid for larger populations, and may also be unreliable for infections that occur in clusters (HIV being an obvious example), where disease rates may vary widely between different communities. Although new clusters indicate a condition whose incidence is changing, they do not in themselves indicate a diseases' 'emergence'. A cluster of cases may be the result of a virulent strain in an immunologically naive population, or of the transmission of infection between contacts, or of an environmental exposure to the same source. Furthermore, publication bias means that while investigators who notice an increase in disease frequency are likely to publish their findings, those who do not notice any change are less likely to publish (Schwartz & Yogev, 1996).

A 1996 study for the WHO and the World Bank entitled *The Global Burden of Disease* reported that infectious diseases accounted for only one of the ten leading causes of death in developed countries – lower respiratory infections was number four on the list and accounted for 3.5 per cent of total deaths. By contrast, infectious diseases (lower respiratory infections, diarrhoeal disease, tuberculosis, measles and malaria) accounted for five of the ten leading causes of deaths and in total account for 26.8 per cent of all deaths in developing countries (Hinman, 1998). Yet even this crude division between developed and developing countries obscures the fact that infectious diseases affect certain developing world countries more than others. In the two poorest regions in the world, sub-Saharan Africa and India, infectious diseases, together with maternal and peri-natal causes of death and nutritional deficiencies, account for the majority of deaths: 65 per cent of deaths in sub-Saharan Africa and 51 per cent of deaths in India. They account for 31 per cent of deaths In Latin America and the Caribbean, 16 per cent of deaths in China, and slightly more than 40 per cent in the other developing regions (Heuveline et al., 2002).

Even a country-by-country analysis obscures the way in which the burden of infectious disease weighs most heavily on the poor, because within both poor and rich countries it is the poorest people who are more likely to succumb to infections. As discussed in Chapter 3, by the late 1980s the idea that AIDS was an exclusively gay disease changed, so the notion that 'everyone was at risk'. Whilst it is true to say that everyone is *potentially* at risk of contracting HIV, it does not mean that everyone is *equally* at risk. EID are portrayed as 'democratic' or 'equal opportunity' illnesses which threaten 'us' all, when in fact the patterns of who is infected and affected by them betray fault lines of social inequality and injustice. The concept of epidemiological transition suggests that as nation states develop they go through predictable epidemiological transformations, so that in richer countries, people are more likely to die of the so-called 'diseases of civilisation'. Yet this model masks the fact that even in the richest countries, the chances of becoming ill or dying prematurely from the 'diseases of civilisation' – cardiovascular disease, diabetes, cancer, even accidents – are inversely related to how rich you are.

This correlation between poverty and increased risk of illness and death is just as valid for infectious diseases as it is for cancer or cardiovascular disease. For example, discussions about the 1918 influenza pandemic frequently cite its death toll of anything between 40 and 100 million people. Yet less often discussed is the variation in mortality rates. In the 1918 outbreak the majority of influenza sufferers recovered within about a week. About 20 per cent developed severe secondary infections that gave rise to fatal pneumonia, sometimes within 24 hours. The deadly complication of influenza pneumonia killed 40 to 50 per cent of people with these secondary infections. Although deaths from TB *decreased* in England and Wales during 1918–19, in the USA, TB mortality peaked along with influenza in 1918. In the USA, co-infection with TB may have contributed to the lethality of the 1918 influenza pandemic because of the synergism between influenza virus and coexisting bacterial infections (Herring, 2009).

The concept of *syndemic* has recently been introduced by medical anthropologists to label such synergistic interaction of two or more coexisting diseases and the resulting excess burden of disease (Singer & Clair, 2003). At its simplest level, and as used by some CDC researchers, the term refers to two or more epidemics interacting synergistically and contributing as a result of their interaction to the burden of disease in a population. For example worldwide, 11 million people are co-infected with both TB and HIV, and TB is the most common HIV-related infection in developing countries. The important point is not just the co-infection with HIV and TB but the enhanced infection due to the interaction of the two diseases. Co-infection reduces the survival time of patients compared with those infected with one or the other as co-infection with HIV and TB can cause reactivation of underlying TB disease. People with HIV may also be more susceptible to infection with TB, and once infected progress more rapidly to disease (Blanc & Uplekar, 2003).

Over and above this sense of *syndemic* as co-infection, the term also points to the sociopolitical context of sufferer's health. Social factors like poverty, stigmatisation, racism, sexism and structural violence (poverty) may be of far greater importance than the nature of pathogens or the bodily systems they infect. Syndemics also involve the interaction of diseases and other adverse health conditions such as malnutrition, substance abuse or stress, as a consequence of health threatening social conditions such as noxious living or working environments. In other words, a syndemic is a set of mutually intertwined and mutually enhancing epidemics involving disease interactions at the biological level that develop and are sustained in a population because of harmful social conditions (Singer & Clair, 2003).

Returning to the 1918 influenza pandemic, the disease also had a disproportionate death toll among young adults, pregnant women, in immigrant and poor neighbourhoods, and in marginalised communities that lacked access to health care. While most national estimates of death rates in 1918–19 ranged between 20 and 50 per 1,000 people, in Europe, influenza mortality rates were lower, ranging from 2.4 per 1,000 in Russia to 12.7 per 1,000 in Hungary. In Canada and the USA they were about six per 1,000. In the Americas, they ranged from 1.2 per 1,000 in Argentina to 39.2 per 1,000 in Guatemala. But in African nations, they ranged from 10.7 per 1,000 people in Egypt to an extraordinarily high 445 per 1,000 in Cameroon (Herring, 2009).

Another example of how the infectious disease burden falls disproportionately on the poor even in the developed world is provided by the re-emergence of TB in NYC in the 1980s. As discussed in Chapter 1, this epidemic was one of the drivers that prompted the creation of the EID category. Yet a resurgence of a disease like TB in an industrialised society does not happen by accident, it requires a massive social upheaval. The TB situation had improved in NYC in the 1960s and 1970s to the point that most new cases were reactivations of latent infections in older people. The root cause of the 're-emergence' of TB was the deliberate destruction of poor neighbourhoods in NYC in the 1970s.

While slum clearance had become legally and politically difficult by the late 1960s, similar aims were achieved in NYC between 1969 and 1976 by a deliberate policy of reducing the fire service in poor, overcrowded neighbourhoods with ageing housing. This resulted in a wave of building fires and a related rise in building abandonment by landlords, with a loss of hundreds of thousands of housing units. Officials gave the impression that a huge proportion of these fires were arson, and thus labelled the slum dwellers as lawless, pathological and antisocial. In fact, less than half of the fires were even suspicious, and proven arson only accounted for a tiny proportion of them. As a result of the social unravelling subsequent to this 'firebombing' of the ghettoes, conditions deteriorated from housing overcrowding and social disruption and about 1.3 million white people left New York. About 0.6 million poor people were displaced and had their homes destroyed. In around five years almost two million people moved, a massive population instability. Effective TB control involves contact tracing and ensuring adherence to medication regimens and is only really possible in stable communities. The re-emergence of TB in NYC in the 1980s was thus a direct consequence of the deliberate policy of de-development. The destruction of housing stock set in motion unintended consequences which spilled out from the ghettos into middle-class neighbourhoods (Wallace & Wallace, 1998; Wallace & Wallace, 2003).

Developing world EID

As in the developed world, in developing countries population-wide averages disguise the way that the burden of infectious diseases bears down most heavily on the poor. In many developing countries, 'epidemiological averages' can seemingly portray a picture of transition towards developed world patterns of morbidity and mortality, giving a misleading impression of population-wide health improvement. However, in effect, the rich and poor, urban and rural dwellers, and other sub-groups of populations in countries may live in different 'epidemiological worlds' (Phillips, 1994).

As discussed in previous chapters, unrestrained *laissez-faire* capitalism and the exploitation of the new industrial urban working class in Europe resulted in nineteenth-century epidemics of classic 'crowd diseases' such as smallpox, tuberculosis and cholera. Similarly, late modern unrestrained economic globalisation has led directly to the emergence of infectious diseases such as HIV/AIDS and re-emergence of older infectious diseases, including TB.

The process by which this came about started with the liberalisation of the global financial markets in the 1970s and 1980s. This led to a far less stable financial system and to poor countries building up debt which they could not repay. Although academics and politicians usually focus on the supposed incompetence of debtor governments and on corruption in poor countries, it was the 'structural adjustments' to developing world economies designed by their creditors, the International Monetary Fund and The World Bank that obliged poor highly indebted nations to repay Northern creditors by diverting money away from improving living standards for their people, including efforts to improve health and tackle infectious diseases (Pettifor, 2006).

For the Victorians, the consequences of the excesses of industrial capitalism and the desperate poverty it caused were present before their very eyes. Today, for most people in developed countries, the wretched poor may now be in 'far-flung' locales, but in a reverse of the 'modernist' belief in progress, the disparities of wealth between the rich and poor are, if anything, growing. For example, at the beginning of the twentieth century, the wealthiest 20 per cent of the world's population were nine times richer than the poorest 20 per cent. That ratio had grown to 30 times richer by 1960, 60 times richer by 1990 and over 80 times richer by 1995. One billion people in the world live well, some in great luxury, while three billion live in poverty. Between 1975 and 1995 the number of extremely poor people in the world doubled. Absolute poverty has also increased more than a quarter of the world's population live on less than US$1 a day. Over half of the 4.4 billion people in developing countries lack access to clean water and essential medicines, and almost a quarter are underfed. As a result of globalised inequalities, there has also arisen a large illicit globalised economy, comprising an illicit arms trade, an illegal drugs trade worth over US$500 billion a year, money laundering, people smuggling, trafficking in endangered species, toxic waste dumping, prostitution, sexual exploitation and child labour (Benatar, 2003).

The slums of early industrialised Europe were known as 'fever nests', but the scale and abject misery of the new developing world mega-slums dwarfs those of Victorian Europe. The British and other colonial powers in Africa, India, Burma and Ceylon built slums and shanty towns on the fringes of segregated cities for the local labour force to live in, resulting in huge death tolls from plague, cholera and influenza in colonial times. Today's developing world slums are the legacy of this colonial urban squalor. The civil wars and political instability of the post-colonial period forced the rural poor to migrate to increasingly overcrowded city slums, where uncollected waste harbours rats and insect vectors like mosquitoes, and where there is no basic sanitation or potable water (Davis, 2006). This type of overcrowding is the most common significant independent predictor of EID, which are found where there are the greater concentrations of people, rather than on the remote fringes of society (Jones et al., 2008).

One of the factors that is said to lead to infectious diseases 'emerging' is changes in agricultural practice. Yet these changes are also a direct result of neoliberal globalisation since the 1980s. In particular they are the result of the reorientation of underdeveloped agricultural subsistence economies towards producing cash crops for export. The forced incorporation of developing world economies into global markets has resulted in the creation of a global class of hungry semi-peasants lacking security of subsistence. Global economic forces that 'push' people from the countryside include the industrial scaling-up and introduction of mechanised agriculture, food imports, and the competition from and the consolidation of smallholdings into larger ones. These changes, combined with population growth and the speed and scale of urbanisation, have led to rising demand in developing countries for poultry, pork and dairy products. This has led to the industrialised mass production of food, the so-called 'livestock revolution', which, like the Green Revolution before it, has favoured corporate mega-producers of food over peasants and family farmers (Davis, 2006).

As discussed in Chapter 5, in light of fears about 'bird flu', mass poultry culls have been carried out in countries across South East Asia. Yet little attention has been paid to the impact of these culls on the food security, nutrition and health of the poor people who bear the brunt of these policies. Chicken is often the cheapest animal protein in developing countries. Over 250 million chickens, mostly from family farms in rural communities, have either died from avian influenza or have been culled in an attempt to stop the spread of the infection. Culling therefore places a large economic burden of farmers who are most vulnerable to economic failures and nutritional inadequacies. Culling poses a threat to families who may only lose a few birds, because these birds represent a measure of food security when shortages in other staples such as fish may occur due to fishing being dangerous during storms (Lockerbie & Herring, 2009).

Similarly, another of the factors often highlighted as causing the emergence of zoonotic infectious diseases, such as HIV, is the supposed African 'fondness' for bushmeat. Yet research into the trade in bushmeat from Ghana demonstrates that increased hunting in nature reserves coincides with years of poor fish supply, the primary source of animal protein consumed in West Africa. Local market data provide evidence of a direct link between poor fish supply and subsequent bushmeat demand – Ghanaians substitute bushmeat for fish because of protein deficiency. Furthermore, declines in fish stocks in West Africa between 1950 and 2000 have coincided with more than tenfold increases in fish harvests in the region by foreign and domestic fishing fleets. The largest foreign presence in West African fisheries is EU boats, which have increased their fishing harvest by a factor of 20 in the same period. Despite declining fish stocks, the EU financial support of its foreign fleet increased from about US$6 million in 1981 to more than US$350 in 2001, significantly and artificially increasing the profitability for EU boats of fishing in African waters (Brashares et al., 2004).

Another of the factors listed as leading to EID 'emerging' is war in and between developing countries. Yet rarely discussed is the relationship between wars and colonial histories, or to the instability caused by economic shock therapy, as discussed above, which have led directly to a rise in insecurity, violence, terrorism and war. Globally there have been 350 wars, revolutions and *coups d'état* since the end of the Second World War, mostly in developing countries (Smallman-Raynor & Cliff, 2003). Modern wars are no longer confrontations between lines of troops, but are more likely to involve civilian populations in close proximity to conflict areas, and civilians and civilian infrastructure such as healthcare facilities are more likely to be seen as legitimate targets. Of those dying in conflict zones, the proportion of civilians has risen from approximately 10 per cent in the First World War to 50 per cent in the Second World War and to 80 per cent in subsequent wars (Weinberg & Simmonds, 1995).

War brings with it mixing of military and civil populations, decreased resistance to infections as a result of physical and mental stress, nutritional deprivation, insanitary conditions, concentration and overcrowding, the interruption of disease control programmes such as immunisation programmes, and the collapse of conventional rules of social behaviour, including rape (Smallman-Raynor & Cliff, 2003). One of the most devastating effects of war is its subsequent forced migration of those refugees fleeing the conflict. In another affront to modernist ideas of 'progress', in 1980, there were 8.4 million people displaced by war, famine and ecological disaster worldwide. By 1992, that number had risen to 17.8 million, and by 2005, the total number of people of concern to the United Nations High Commission for Refugees (UNHCR) was 19.2 million (Pettifor, 2006).

TB, MDR-TB and HIV/AIDS

The decontextualisation of the 'factors' causing infectious diseases to 'emerge' from their social, economic and political causes is nowhere more evident than in discussions of the 're-emergence' of TB. Nearly one-third of the world's population – two billion people – is infected with the tuberculosis bacterium and at risk of developing the disease. About eight million people develop active TB every year, and two million die, of which some 95 per cent of cases and 98 per cent of deaths are in the developing world. In much of the world, TB is the leading killer of young adults, in spite of effective treatments being available for the past 50 years. As well as this holocaust of entirely preventable illness and premature death, the economic costs of TB to patients and their families can be crippling, as they not only lose income due to inability to work, but also have to liquidise whatever meagre assets they may have in order to pay for treatment (Blanc & Uplekar, 2003).

The 'conquest' of TB is one of the heroic narratives of the 'golden age of medicine'. Yet as the anthropologist and medical doctor Paul Farmer has argued passionately, although there have been dramatic shifts in local TB epidemiology in certain populations, a more global analysis does not suggest there has been major decreases in TB as a cause of death. The invisibility of the disease in the 1970s and 1980s relates to disease awareness – TB did not 're-emerge' so much as emerge from the ranks of the poor. In spite of theoretical risks to the 'general population' the majority of US cases of TB remain among the inner-city poor, in prisons, homeless shelters and public hospitals. The 're-emergence' of 'new' TB is a result of global social and economic changes, which has led to mass movements of people in response to war, economic insecurity and community breakdown, spreading TB and other infectious diseases in overcrowded and makeshift housing (Gandy, 2003).

In response to the rise in transmission of TB and outbreaks of multi-drug-resistant TB (MDR-TB) associated with HIV, the Global Project on Drug Resistance was launched in 1994 to monitor trends. Between 1997 and 2000, reports showed that drug resistance was present worldwide and the prevalence of MDR-TB ranged from 0 to 14 per cent of new cases (median 1.4 per cent) and 0 to 54 per cent of cases of previously treated cases (median 13 per cent). Between 1999 and 2002 there were decreases in MDR-TB prevalence in Hong Kong, Thailand and the USA, but significant increases in Estonia, Lithuania, Russia and Poland. Most western and central European states only see a few cases of MDR-TB each year, but two Chinese provinces, Henan and Hubei, saw more than 1000 cases each year, and Kazakhstan and South Africa have more than 3000 cases each (Victor & Young, 2005).

Biomedical publications often talk of MDR-TB being the result of 'sub-optimal dosage' and 'poor drug absorption' while remaining coy about why people take their anti-TB medication erratically, or ignoring the issue of lack of access to optimal treatment in poor communities in the USA and elsewhere. Often social scientists talk of non-adherence to therapies being the result of 'behavioural problems', or anthropologists of 'health beliefs' 'sorcery' or 'folk beliefs'. The effect of poverty on people's ability to receive effective treatment is less often mentioned. In most places, the degree to which patients are able to comply with their TB treatment regimens is significantly limited by forces outside of their control (Farmer, 1997).

Just as the re-emergence of TB in NYC in the 1980s followed a massive social upheaval in the city, so the re-emergence of TB in the post-Soviet bloc countries was also caused directly by the social disruption and capital flight that accompanied the end of the communist era. In the Soviet era, TB care was organised, and there were programmes for BCG vaccination and mass TB screening programmes. As a result, by the 1970s, instances of TB were rare. By 1989, just at the end of the Soviet era, the TB rate was 44.7 per 100,000. Yet by 1998, the TB rates were 81.3 per 100,000 for Latvia, 82.4 for the Russian Federation, 89.1 for Turkmenistan 96.4 for Georgia, 114 for Romania, 122.9 for Kyrgyzstan and 126.4 for Kazakhstan (Stern, 2003). In the 1990s, using the money they had sequestered during the 'privatisation' of former Soviet assets, the new Russian super-rich oligarchs hugely inflated prices of luxury housing in London and elsewhere. Meanwhile the economies of the former Soviet countries dramatically unravelled. As a result, millions of people who had previously maintained a moderate standard of living found themselves abruptly plunged into poverty.

The economic crisis in the former Soviet Union led to massive social disruption, a sudden increase in crime and a consequent increase in the prison population. By 2000, the Russian Federation had imprisonment rates of 678 per 100,000, the second highest in the world after the USA at 682 per 100,000. (By comparison, southern Europe's median rate is 70 and in England and Wales it is 125.) In 1998, a Moscow press conference organised by three NGOs announced that 100,000 prisoners, one in ten of the Russian prisoner population, suffered from active TB, and 20,000 had MDR-TB (Stern, 2003). Russian prisoners were developing MDR-TB as a result of ineffective treatment of the strains of TB which were resistant to the drugs being administered to them. Various observers, including some from international human rights organisations, argued that these prisoners have 'untreatable forms' of TB, although treatment based on the standard of care expected elsewhere in Europe and North America would cure the vast majority of these cases. 'Untreatable' in this context means 'too expensive to treat' (Farmer, 2005).

It has been said that the impact of the syndemic of HIV/AIDS and TB in South Africa within the next five to 20 years may reduce the country to widespread social anarchy – a society reduced to living out the values of a movie gangland dystopia such as that portrayed in the movie *Mad Max* (Shell, 2000 in Brower & Chalk, 2003). South Africa is now listed by the WHO as one of the highest burdened countries in terms of MDR-TB. In fact, MDR-TB was first identified in South Africa, in the Western Cape area, in 1985. By 1994, MDR-TB accounted for 2 per cent of TB in the region (Victor & Young, 2005). Just as the re-emergence of TB in NYC was the unintended but direct result of racist housing policies in the city, so South Africa's TB and HIV/AIDS syndemic, the worst in the world, is also a direct consequence of generations of racist government policies there.

The history of TB in South Africa dates back to the discovery of diamonds and gold there in the 1880s. This led to a rapid urbanisation of Africans, and a devastating epidemic of TB, as Africans came into contact with infected European immigrants in overcrowded slums. As a result of a lack of medical attention, overcrowding in slums and a poor diet, Africans either succumbed to TB, or survived to becoming reservoirs of infection for others. Sick migrant workers were repatriated to rural areas, infecting others who subsequently migrated to urban areas carrying with them latent TB infections. In the 1920s and 1930s South Africa's TB policy was to exclude and segregate cases through slum clearance, rather than dealing with the underlying causes. In the late 1930s and 1940s, there was a new wave of TB disease amongst blacks, which by 1945 led to white public hysteria about the threat to both labour supply and to the health of whites (Packard, 1989).

The victory of the South African National Party in 1948 marked the beginning of an era marked by dramatic changes in the epidemiology of TB in South Africa. Although urban TB mortality rates began to fall in response to new treatments, between 1948 and 1985 there was little or no amelioration of the underlying causes of TB. Millions of Africans were forcibly moved to already overcrowded reservations. The residents of the new townships had to travel long distances to work on overcrowded public transport, exposing them to the risk of TB infection. The inequitable distribution of health services in South Africa, combined with the pattern of racial segregation, decreased the likelihood that black TB cases would be effectively cured, and increased the numbers of partially cured cases who would be a source of infection to others. So even before the impact of HIV/AIDS in the 1990s, the TB rates in urban South Africa were already extremely high. Between 1979 and 1989 over 25,000 people died of TB in South Africa, nearly all of whom were Africans, coloureds and Asians. In 1989, white cases made up only one per cent of new cases each year (Packard, 1989). HIV/AIDS undoubtedly contributed to the TB epidemic in South Africa, as it did in certain US and European cities. Yet HIV/AIDS did not cause TB to 're-emerge'. In developed and developing countries, the 're-emergence' of TB had begun long before HIV had penetrated poor communities.

The fact that the HIV/AIDS epidemic is worse in sub-Saharan Africa than anywhere else in the world is usually blamed on African sexuality, prostitution, ignorance and corruption, rather than on unrestrained globalised capitalism, exploitation and racism. African sexuality is often portrayed as rooted in 'traditional' African culture, and thus difficult to change. Yet contemporary African sexual mores are, at least in part, a legacy of colonial racist policies. As discussed above, the colonial powers needed cheap African labour for activities such as mining and construction. At the same time, so that they would not have any claims on urban land, African migrant workers were denied permission to bring their families with them. One effect of this was the breakdown of traditional rules and protocols of marriage, leading to unprecedented inter-ethnic (transient and longer-lasting) sexual relationships and marriages (Aina, 1988).

This brings us back to the discussion in Chapter 3 and to the questions posed in the debate around AIDS in the late 1980s: Why was there a HIV/AIDS epidemic amongst gay men in the West, yet the predicted Western heterosexual epidemic did not materialise? And, conversely, why is there such a catastrophic HIV epidemic amongst heterosexuals in certain countries in sub-Saharan Africa but not elsewhere?

The reason why gay men are disproportionately at risk of contracting HIV is often assumed to be as a result of anal sex. As discussed in Chapter 3, the widespread belief is that because the anus was not 'designed' for penetration, it is less 'rugged' than a vagina, and thus more at risk of tearing, and hence HIV transmission. Yet while unprotected anal sex may be slightly more dangerous than unprotected vaginal sex in terms of the likelihood of HIV transmission, unprotected vaginal sex is still a perfectly efficient way of passing on the HIV virus, as the experience in sub-Saharan Africa and elsewhere demonstrates. The reason why gay men are more 'at risk' of contracting HIV relates not to anal sex, but to patterns of partner change.

The model for sexual partner change amongst modern Western heterosexuals is slow serial monogamy. This heterosexual model is bolstered by legally binding and socially sanctioned marriage, and by extension the societal recognition of long-term unmarried heterosexual partnerships. AIDS affects both Africans and gay men disproportionately, something often 'explained' away with the word 'promiscuity', without giving any social context of why that might be the case. When HIV was spreading through the gay communities of Europe and North America in the 1970s and 1980s, the same social forces that keep heterosexual couples together were pushing in the opposite direction, away from the possibility of gay men forming stable relationships. The strength of continuing opposition to 'gay marriage' in many Western countries, such as Italy and the USA, illustrates the discrimination and homophobia that formed, and still forms, the background to many gay men's lived experience.

The 'promiscuity' of gay men and Africans is at least in part a product of a set of particular social circumstances, rather than something 'natural', 'cultural' or a taken-for-granted 'fact'. With the exception of people infected by blood products or transfusions, what all people affected by HIV have in common is their marginalised status: whether as a result of their sexual orientation, of poverty, and in some societies their ethnicity or gender (Pisani, 2008).

The idea that 'everyone is at risk of AIDS' is therefore only true in about 3 per cent of the world. Patterns of sexual partner change account for the fact that for many years now, most new HIV infections in Asia, Europe, the Americas, Australasia, the Middle East, North Africa and even parts of West Africa are either the result of sex between men, drug use, or amongst people who buy and sell sex (Pisani, 2008). The difference between Africa and the rest of the world in terms of HIV transmission is that in much of East and Southern Africa heterosexuals, like some Western gay men, have sex with networks of people, often regular partners, but who themselves may also be having sex with more than one regular partner.

The burden of infectious disease falls disproportionately on the poor, particularly, though not exclusively, poor people in the developing world. Yet the discourse around EID is itself rarely contextualised in terms of the burden of other infectious diseases left outside the 'emerging or re-emerging' category (because they do not threaten people in the developed world). AIDS kills about one million people a year, but malaria has a similar death toll. Yet malaria is thought of not as an 'emerging' disease, but rather as 'endemic' in the developing world. Malaria only registers in the EID discourse in terms of the discussion of global warming, with fears that malaria may 'emerge' in 'our' part of the world. AIDS is an 'emerging' disease insofar as it is new, yet the context of AIDS in Africa is that 50 per cent of Africa's population would have died before the age of forty even without AIDS, while in Western Europe and Japan 50 per cent of the population will live past 80 (Alcabes, 2009).

On many levels, the late modern discourse about the risk of EID echoes the arguments that were being made in the earlier industrial era, and which led to the modern public health movement. Infectious diseases thrive in conditions of poverty, social exclusion and inequality. Part of the thinking behind the EID worldview is to motivate rich countries to improve infectious disease control and surveillance through enlightened self-interest. But in order to stop infectious diseases from emerging and re-emerging, we cannot simply draw up the bridges by which they travel from the poor to the rich. Exclusion in itself will never be sufficient to prevent or contain EID, even supposing that such a strategy would be possible in our globalised world. In order to really stem EID we would need to start by distributing the world's resources more fairly, and to tackle the discrimination, homophobia and racism that blight so many lives. These are the factors that lead, directly and indirectly, to the emergence and re-emergence of infectious diseases.

References

Ahmad, D. (2000). Opium smoking, anti-Chinese attitudes, and the American medical community, 1850–1890. *American Nineteenth Century History*, 1, 53–68.

Aina, T. (1988). The myth of African promiscuity. In R. Sabatier (ed.), *Blaming Others: Prejudice, Race and Worldwide AIDS*. London: The Panos Institute, pp. 76–8.

Alcabes, P. (2009). *Dread: How Fear and Fantasy Have Fueled Epidemics from the Black Death to Avian Flu*. New York: Public Affairs.

Allen, S. (2002). *Media, Risk and Science*. Buckingham: Open University Press.

Altman, D. (1986). *AIDS and the New Puritanism*. London: Pluto Press.

Altman, S. & over 700 additional signatories (2005). An open letter to Elias Zerhouni. *Science*, 307, 1409–10.

Anderson, W. (1996). Immunities of Empire: Race, disease, and the new tropical medicine, 1900–1920. *Bulletin of the History of Medicine*, 70, 94–118.

Annas, G. (2003). Terrorism and human rights. In J. Moreno (ed.), *In the Wake of Terror: Medicine and Morality in a Time of Crisis*. Cambridge, MA: The MIT Press, pp. 33–51.

Armelagos, G., Brown, P. & Turner, B. (2005). Evolutionary, historical and political perspectives on health and disease. *Social Science & Medicine*, 61, 755–65.

Ashenberg, K. (2007). *Clean: An Unsanitised History of Washing*. London: Profile Books.

Ashraf, H. (2002). Bioterror and HIV dominate infectious disease meeting. *The Lancet*, 360, 1076.

Ayliffe, G. & English, M. (2003). *Hospital Infection: From Miasmas to MRSA*. Cambridge: Cambridge University Press.

Baehr, P. (2006). Susan Sontag, battle language and the Hong Kong SARS outbreak of 2003. *Economy and Society*, 35, 42–64.

Barber, B. (1995). *Jihad vs. McWorld: Terrorism's Challenge to Democracy*. New York: Random House.

Barde, R. (2003). Prelude to the plague: Public health and politics at America's Pacific gateway, 1899. *Journal of the History of Medicine*, 58, 153–86.

Barker, M. (1981). *The New Racism: Conservatives and the Ideology of the Tribe*. London: Junction Books.

Barrett, R., Kuzawa, C.W., McDade, T., & Armelagos, G.J. (1998). Emerging and re-emerging infectious diseases: The third epidemiologic transition. *Annual Review of Anthropology*, 27, 247–71.

Barry, J. (2005). *The Great Influenza: The Epic Story of the Deadliest Plague in History*. London: Penguin Books.

Bayer, R. & Colgrove, J. (2003). Rights and dangers: Bioterrorism and the ideologies of public health. In J. Moreno (ed.), *In the Wake of Terror: Medicine and Morality in a Time of Crisis*. Cambridge, MA: The MIT Press, pp. 51–75.

Beck, U. (1986). *Risk Society: Towards a New Modernity*. London: Sage Publications.

Beck, U. (2000). *What is Globalisation?* Cambridge: Polity Press.

Beck, U. (2006). Living in the world risk society. A Hobhouse memorial lecture given at the London School of Economics and Political Science. *Economy and Society*, 35, 329–45.

Bell, M., Brown, T., & Faire, L. (2006). Germs, genes and postcolonial geographies: Reading the return of tuberculosis to Leicester, UK, 2001. *Cultural Geographies*, 13, 577–99.

Benatar, S. (2003). Global poverty and tuberculosis: Implications for ethics and human rights. In M. Gandy & A. Zumla (eds), *The Return of the White Plague: Global Poverty and the 'New' Tuberculosis*. London: Verso, pp. 222–36.

Bengtsson, T. (1999). The vulnerable child. Economic insecurity and child mortality in pre-industrial Sweden: A case study. *European Journal of Population*, 15, 117–51.

Berkelman, R. & Freeman, P. (2004). Emerging infections and the CDC response. In R. Packard, P. Brown, R. Berkelman & H. Frumkin (eds), *Emerging Illness and Society: Negotiating the Public Health Agenda*. Baltimore and London: The Johns Hopkins University Press, pp. 350–88.

Bhattacharjee, Y. (2008). FBI to request scientific review of its anthrax investigation. *Science*, 916, 1.

Blanc, L. & Uplekar, M. (2003). The present global burden of tuberculosis. In M. Gandy & A. Zumla (eds), *The Return of the White Plague: Global Poverty and the 'New' Tuberculosis*. London: Verso, pp. 95–111.

Blendon, R., Benson, J., DesRoches, C., Raleigh, E., & Taylor-Clark, K. (2004). The public's response to the severe acute respiratory syndrome in Toronto and the United States. *Clinical Infectious Diseases*, 38, 925–31.

Blumberg, B. (1977). Australia antigen and the biology of hepatitis B. *Science*, 197, 17–25.

Blumberg, B. (1988). Hepatitis B virus and the carrier problem. *Social Research*, 55, 401–12.

Blume, S. (2006). Anti-vaccination movements and their interpretations. *Social Science & Medicine*, 62, 628–42.

Bonanni, P. (1999). Demographic impact of vaccination: A review. *Vaccine*, 17, S125.

Booth, K. (2000). 'Just testing'. Race, sex and the media in New York's 'baby AIDS' debate. *Gender and Society*, 14, 644–61.

Boyce, T., Swedlow, D. & Griffin, P. (1996). Shiga toxin-producing *Escherichia coli* infections and hemolytic uremic syndrome. *Seminars in Pediatric Infectious Diseases*, 7, 258–64.

Boylston, A. (2002). Clinical investigation of smallpox in 1767. *New England Journal of Medicine*, 346, 1326–8.

Brandt, A. (1985). *No Magic Bullet: A Social History of Venereal Disease in the United States since 1880*. Oxford: Oxford University Press.

Brandt, A. (1988). AIDS and metaphor: Toward the social meaning of epidemic disease. *Social Research*, 55, 413–32.

Brashares, J., Arcese, P., Moses, K., Coppolillo, P., Sinclair, A. & Balmford, A. (2004). Bushmeat hunting, wildlife declines, and fish supply in West Africa. *Science*, 306, 1180–3.

Breugelmans, J., Zucs, P., Porten, K., Broll, S., Niedrig, M., Ammon, A. et al. (2004). SARS transmission and commercial aircraft. *Emerging Infectious Diseases*, 10, 1502–3.

Broadway, M. (2008). The social representation and reality of BSE's impact in North Central Alberta. *The Canadian Geographer*, 52, 451–65.

Brookes, R. (1999). Newspapers and national identity: The BSE/CJD crisis in the British press. *Media Culture Society*, 21, 247–63.

Brower, J. & Chalk, P. (2003). *The Global Threat of New and Reemerging Infectious Diseases: Reconciling US National Security and Public Health Policy*. Santa Monica, CA: RAND Corporation.

Brown, D. (1996). The 1990 Florida dental investigation: Theory and fact. *Annals of Internal Medicine*, 124, 255–6.

Bud, R. (1978). Strategy in American cancer research after World War II: A case study. *Social Studies of Science*, 8, 425–59.

Bud, R. (1998). Penicillin and the new Elizabethans. *British Journal for the History of Science*, 31, 305–33.

Bud, R. (2006). *Penicillin: Triumph and the Tragedy*. Oxford: Oxford University Press.

Buus, S. & Olsson, E. (2006). The SARS crisis: Was anyone responsible? *The Journal of Contingencies and Crisis Management*, 12, 71–81.

Campkin, B. (2007). Degradation and regeneration: Theories of dirt and the contemporary city. In B. Campkin & R. Cox (eds), *Dirt: New Geographies of Cleanliness and Contamination*. London and New York: IB Tauris, pp. 68–80.

Campkin, B. & Cox, R. (2007). Materialities and metaphors of dirt and cleanliness. In B. Campkin & R. Cox (eds), *Dirt: New Geographies of Cleanliness and Contamination*. London and New York: IB Tauris, pp. 1–11.

Cannon, G. (1995). *Superbug: Nature's Revenge. Why Antibiotics can Breed Disease*. London: Virgin Publishing.

Cantor, N. (2001). *In the Wake of the Plague: The Black Death and the World it Made*. London: Pocket Books.

Carson, R. (1962). *Silent Spring*. New York: Fawcett Spring.

CDC (1981). Pneumocystis Pneumonia – Los Angeles. *MMWR Weekly*, 30, 250–2.

CDC (1987). Epidemiologic notes and reports update: Human immunodeficiency virus infections in health-care workers exposed to blood of infected patients. *MMWR Weekly*, 36, 285–9.

CDC (1994). *Addressing Emerging Infectious Disease Threats: A Prevention Strategy for the United States*. Atlanta: Center for Disease Control.

CDC (1998). *Preventing Emerging Infectious Diseases: A Strategy for the 21st Century*. Atlanta: Center for Disease Control.

CDC (2001). STDs among men who have sex with men. *STD Surveillance – Special Focus Profiles, 2001*, 65–9.

Chavers, S., Fawal, H. & Vermund, S. (2002). An introduction to emerging and reemerging infectious diseases. In F. Lashley & J. Durham (eds), *Emerging Infectious Diseases: Trends and Issues*. New York: Springer Publishing Company, pp. 3–22.

Chen, L. & Narasimhan, V. (2003). Human security and global health. *Journal of Human Development and Capabilities*, 4, 181–90.

Chiang, W. & Duann, R. (2007). Conceptual metaphors for SARS: 'War' between whom? *Discourse and Society*, 18, 579–602.

Childers, J. (2005). Foreign matter: Imperial filth. In W. Cohen & R. Johnson (eds), *Filth: Dirt, Disgust and Modern Life*. Minneapolis: University of Minnesota Press, pp. 201–24.

Childress, J. (2003). Triage in response to a bioterrorist attack. In J. Moreno (ed.), *In the Wake of Terror: Medicine and Morality in a Time of Crisis*. Cambridge, MA: The MIT Press, pp. 77–95.

Chirimuuta, R. & Chirimuuta, R. (1987). *AIDS Africa and Racism*. Derbyshire: Bretby.

Chubin, D. & Studer, K. (1978). The politics of cancer. *Theory and Society*, 6, 55–74.

Clarke, L., Chess, C., Holmes, R. & O'Neill, K. (2006). Speaking with one voice: Risk communication lessons from the US anthrax attacks. *Journal of Contingencies and Crisis Management*, 14, 160–9.

Classen, C., Howes, D., & Synnott, A. (1994). *Aroma: The Cultural History of Smell*. London and New York: Routledge.

Cliff, A. & Haggett, P. (2004). Time, travel and infection. *British Medical Bulletin*, 69, 87–99.

Cockburn, A. (1963). *The Evolution and Eradication of Infectious Diseases*. Baltimore: The Johns Hopkins Press.

Cohen, W. (2005). Locating filth. In W. Cohen & R. Johnson (eds), *Filth: Dirt, Disgust and Modern Life*. Minneapolis: University of Minnesota Press.

Collinge, J. (1999). Variant Creutzfeldt-Jacob disease. *The Lancet*, 354, 317–23.

Committee on Smallpox Vaccination Program Implementation (2005). *The Smallpox Vaccination Program: Public Health in an Age of Terrorism*. Washington, DC: The National Academies Press.

Corbin, A. (1986). *The Foul and the Fragrant: Odor and the French Social Imagination*. Leamington Spa: Berg.

Craddock, S. (1995). Sewers and scapegoats: Spatial metaphors of smallpox in nineteenth century San Francisco. *Social Science & Medicine*, 41, 957–68.

Craddock, S. (1998). Tuberculosis, tenements and the epistemology of neglect: San Francisco in the nineteenth century. *ECUMENE*, 5, 53–80.

Crawford, D. (2007). *Deadly Companions: How Microbes Shaped our History*. Oxford: Oxford University Press.

Cyranoski, D. (2001). Outbreak of chicken flu rattles Hong Kong. *Nature*, 412, 261.

Danzig, R. & Berkowsky, P. (1999). Why should we be concerned about biological warfare? In J. Lederberg (ed.), *Biological Weapons: Limiting the Threat*. Cambridge, MA: The MIT Press, pp. 9–14.

Davey, C. (2002). Hepatitis C. In F. Lashley & J. Durham (eds), *Emerging Infectious Diseases: Trends and Issues*. New York: Springer Publishing Company, pp. 151–60.

David, M. (2005). *Science in Society*. Basingstoke: Palgrave Macmillan.

Davis, M. (2005). *The Monster at our Door: The Global Threat of Avian Flu*. New York and London: The New Press.

Davis, M. (2006). *Planet of Slums*. London and New York: Verso.

Dealler, S. (1996). *Lethal Legacy. BSE: The Search for the Truth*. London: Bloomsbury Publishing.

Delaney, M. (2000). HIV, AIDS, and the distortion of science. *Focus*, 15, 1–6.

Demko, V. (1998). An analysis of media coverage of the BSE crisis in the United States. In S. Razan (ed.), *The Mad Cow Crisis: Health and the Public Good*. London: UCL Press, pp. 153–66.

Deng, I., Duku, O., Gillo, A., Idris, A., Lolik, P., el Tahir, B. et al. (1978). Ebola haemorrhagic fever in Sudan, 1976. Report of a WHO/International study team. *Bulletin of the World Health Organization*, 56, 247–70.

Department of Health (2004). *Towards Cleaner Hospitals and Lower Rates of Infection: A Summary of Action*. London: HMSO.

Dew, K. (1999). Epidemics, panic and power: Representations of measles and measles vaccines. *Health*, 3, 379–98.

Dismukes, W. (1996). Emerging and reemerging infections. *The American Journal of Medicine*, 100, 12–14.

Douglas, M. (1966). *Purity and Danger: An Analysis of Concepts of Pollution and Taboo*. London: Routledge and Kegan Paul Ltd.

Douglas, M. (1992). *Risk and Blame*. London: Routledge.

Douglas, M. & Wildavsky, A. (1982). *Risk and Culture: An Essay on the Selection of Technological and Environmental Dangers*. Berkeley and Los Angeles: University of California Press.

Dubos, R. (1959). *Mirage of Health: Utopias, Progress and Biological Change*. New Brunswick and London: Rutgers University Press.

Dubos, R. & Dubos, J. (1952). *The White Plague: Tuberculosis, Man and Society*. New Brunswick, NJ: Rutgers University Press.

Duerden, B. (2007). Confronting infection in the English National Health Service. *Journal of Hospital Infection*, 65, 23–6.

Eckenwiler, L. (2003). Emergency health professionals and the ethics of crisis. In J. Moreno (ed.), *In the Wake of Terror: Medicine and Morality in a Time of Crisis*. Cambridge, MA: The MIT Press, pp. 111–33.

Eichelberger, L. (2007). SARS and New York's Chinatown: The politics of risk and blame during an epidemic of fear. *Social Science & Medicine*, 65, 1284–95.

Elbe, S. (2008). Our epidemiological footprint: The circulation of avian flu, SARS, and HIV/AIDS in the world economy. *Review of International Political Economy*, 15, 116–30.

Eldridge, J., Kitzinger, J., & Williams, K. (1997). *The Mass Media and Power in Modern Britain*. Oxford: Oxford University Press.

Elias, N. (1939). *The Civilising Process*. (1994 ed.) Oxford: Blackwell Publishing.

Ellis, W. & Lashley, F. (2002). Ebola, Marburg and Lassa fevers. In F. Lashley & J. Durham (eds), *Emerging Infectious Diseases: Trends and Issues*. New York: Springer Publishing Company, pp. 113–28.

Enserink, M. (2008). Anthrax Investigation: Full-Genome Sequencing Paved the Way From Spores to a Suspect. *Science*, 321, 898–9.

Enserink, M. & Kaiser, J. (2005). Has biodefense gone overboard? *Science*, 307, 1396–8.

Fairchild, A. (2004). Policies of inclusion: Immigrants, disease, dependency, and American immigration policy at the dawn and dusk of the 20th century. *American Journal of Public Health*, 94, 528–39.

Fairchild, A. & Tynan, E. (1994). Policies of containment: Immigration in the era of AIDS. *American Journal of Public Health*, 84, 2011–22.

Farmer, P. (1997). Social scientists and the new tuberculosis. *Social Science and Medicine*, 44, 347–58.

Farmer, P. (1999). *Infections and Inequalities: The Modern Plagues*. Berkeley and Los Angeles: University of California Press.

Farmer, P. (2005). *Pathologies of Power: Health, Human Rights and the New War on the Poor*. Berkeley and Los Angeles: University of California Press.

Farrar, J. & Adegbola, R. (2005). Vietnam and the Gambia: Antibiotic resistance in developing countries. In G. Newton (ed.), *Antibiotic Resistance: An Unwinnable War?* London: The Wellcome Trust, pp. 32–4.

Fauci, A. (2006). *Emerging and Re-emerging Infectious Diseases: The Perpetual Challenge* 2005 Robert H Ebert Memorial Lecture. Milbank Memorial Fund. Available: www.milbank.org/reports/0601Fauci/0601Fauci.html.

Feldberg, G. (2006). Making history: TB and the public health legacy of SARS in Canada. In J. Duffin & A. Sweetman (eds), *SARS in Context: Memory, History, Policy*. Montreal: McGill-Queens University Press, pp. 105–20.

Fenner, F., Henderson, D.A., Arita, I., Jezec, Z., & Ladnyi, I. (1988). *Smallpox and its Eradication*. Geneva: World Health Organization.

Ferguson, J. (1999). Biological weapons and the US law. In J. Lederberg (ed.), *Biological Weapons: Limiting the Threat*. Cambridge, MA: The MIT Press, pp. 81–92.

Fisher, J.A. (1994). *The Plague Makers*. New York: Simon and Schuster.

Foucault, M. (1973). *The Birth of the Clinic*. London: Routledge.

Fry, A. & Besser, R. (2002). Legionellosis: Legionnaires' disease and Pontiac fever. In F. Lashley & J. Durham (eds), *Emerging Infectious Diseases: Trends and Issues*. New York: Springer Publishing Company, pp. 171–80.

Gainer, B. (1972). *The Alien Invasion: The Origins of the Aliens Act of 1905*. London: Heinemann Educational Books.

Gandy, M. (2003). Life without germs: Contested episodes in the history of tuberculosis. In M. Gandy & A. Zumla (eds), *The Return of the White Plague: Global Poverty and the 'New' Tuberculosis*. London: Verso, pp. 15–39.

Gardner, D. (2008). *Risk: The Science and Politics of Fear*. London: Virgin Books.

Garrett, L. (1995). *The Coming Plague: Newly Emerging Diseases in a World out of Balance*. New York: Penguin.

Garrett, L. (2001). The nightmare of bioterrorism. *Foreign Affairs*, 80, 76–89.

Giddens, A. (1990). *The Consequences of Modernity*. Cambridge: Polity Press.

Giddens, A. (1991). *Modernity and Self-Identity*. Stanford: Stanford University Press.

Gieger, H. (2001). Terrorism, biological weapons, and bonanzas: Assessing the real threat to public health. *American Journal of Public Health*, 91, 708–9.

Gilbert, P. (2005). Medical mapping: The Thames, the body and *Our Mutual Friend*. In W. Cohen & R. Johnson (eds), *Filth: Dirt, Disgust and Modern Life*. Minneapolis: University of Minnesota Press, pp. 78–102.

Goldacre, B. (2008). *Bad Science*. London: Harper Perennial.

Goozner, M (2003, 30 September). Bioterror brain drain. *The American Prospect*. Available: www.prospect.org/cs/articles?article=bioterror_brain_drain.

Gostin, L., Sapsin, J., Teret, S., Burris, S., Mair, J., Hodge, J. et al. (2002). The Model State Emergency Health Powers Act: Planning for and response to bioterrorim and naturally occurring infectious diseases. *Journal of the American Medical Association*, 288, 622–8.

Gottlieb, M. (2001). AIDS – Past and future. *New England Journal of Medicine*, 344, 1788–91.

Gottlieb, M., Schanker, H., Fan, P., Saxon, A. & Weisman, J. (1981). Pneumocystis pneumonia – Los Angeles. *New England Journal of Medicine*, 305, 1425–31.

Gould, T. (1995). *A Summer Plague: Polio and its Survivors.* New Haven and London: Yale University Press.

Grant, W. (1997). BSE and the politics of food. In P. Dunleavy (ed.), *Developments in British Politics.* Basingstoke: Macmillan, pp. 342–54.

Gregory, J. & Miller, J. (1998). *Science in Public: Communication, Culture and Credibility.* New York and London: Plenum Trade.

Groom, A. & Cheek, J. (2002). Hantavirus pulmonary syndrome. In F. Lashley & J. Durham (eds), *Emerging Infectious Diseases: Trends and Issues.* New York: Springer Publishing Company, pp. 139–50.

Guillemin, J. (1999). *Anthrax: The Investigation of a Deadly Outbreak.* Berkeley: University of California Press.

Gwyn, R. (1999). 'Killer bugs', 'silly buggers' and 'politically correct pals': Competing discourses in health scare reporting. *Health*, 3, 335–45.

Haggett, P. (1994). Geographical aspects of the emergence of infectious diseases. *Geografiska Annaler Series B, Human Geography*, 76, 91–104.

Hahn, B. & Shaw, G. (2000). AIDS as a zoonosis: Scientific and public health implications. *Science*, 287, 607–14.

Hardy, A. (1993). *The Epidemic Streets. Infectious Disease and the Rise of Preventative Medicine 1856–1900.* Oxford: Clarendon Press.

Henderson, D.A. (1999). About the first national symposium on medical and public health response to bioterrorism. *Emerging Infectious Diseases*, 5, 491.

Henderson, D.A. & Fenner, F. (2001). Recent events and observations pertaining to smallpox virus destruction in 2002. *Clinical Infectious Diseases*, 33, 1057–9.

Henretig, F. (2001). Biological and chemical terrorism defense: A view from the 'front lines' of public health. *American Journal of Public Health*, 91, 718–20.

Herring, D. (2009). Viral panic, vulnerability and the next pandemic. In C. Panter-Brick & A. Fuentes (eds), *Health, Risk, and Adversity: A Contextual View from Anthropology.* Oxford: Berghahn Press, pp. 78–97.

Herzlich, C. & Pierret, J. (1984). *Illness and Self in Society.* Baltimore and London: John Hopkins Press.

Herzlich, C. & Pierret, J. (1989). The construction of a social phenomenon: AIDS in the French press. *Social Science and Medicine*, 29, 1235–42.

Heuveline, P., Guillot, M. & Gwatkin, R. (2002). The uneven tides of health transition. *Social Science and Medicine*, 55, 322.

Hewitt, J. & Schmid, M. (2002). Cryptosporidiosis. In F. Lashley & J. Durham (eds), *Emerging Infectious Diseases: Trends and Issues.* New York: Springer Publishing Company, pp. 83–92.

Hewlett, B. & Amola, P. (2003). Cultural contexts of Ebola in northern Uganda. *Emerging Infectious Diseases*, 9, 1242–8.

Heymann, D. (2003). The evolving infectious disease threat: Implications for national and global security. *Journal of Human Development and Capabilities*, 4, 191–207.

Hillis, D. (2000). Origins of HIV. *Science*, 288, 1757–9.

Hinchliffe, S. (2000). Living with risk: The unnatural geography of environmental crises. In S. Hinchliffe & K. Woodward (eds), *The Natural and the Social: Uncertainty, Risk and Change.* London and New York: Routledge, pp. 117–54.

Hinman, A. (1998). Global progress in infectious disease control. *Vaccine*, 16, 1116–21.

Hodge, J. & Gostin, L. (2003). Protecting the public's health in an era of bioterrorism: The model State Emergency Health Powers Act. In J. Moreno (ed.), *In the Wake of Terror: Medicine and Morality in a Time of Crisis.* Cambridge, MA: The MIT Press, pp. 17–33.

Holtzclaw, B. (2002). Dengue fever. In F. Lashley & J. Durham (eds), *Emerging Infectious Diseases: Trends and Issues.* New York: Springer Publishing Company, pp. 103–12.

Hui, E. (2006). Reasons for the increase in emerging and re-emerging viral infectious diseases. *Microbes and Infection,* 8, 905–16.

Huminer, D., Rosenfeld, J., & Pitlik, S. (1987). AIDS in the pre-AIDS era. *Reviews of Infectious Diseases,* 9, 1102–8.

Ibrahim, M. (2005). The securitization of migration: A racial discourse. *International Migration,* 43, 163–87.

Illich, I. (1976). *Limits to Medicine. Medical Nemesis: The Expropriation of Health.* London: Marion Boyars.

Ingram, A. (2005). The new geopolitics of disease: Between global health and global security. *Geopolitics,* 10, 522–45.

Ingram, A. (2007). HIV/AIDS, security and the geopolitics of US–Nigerian relations. *Review of International Political Economy,* 14, 510–34.

James, S. & Sargent, T. (2006). The economic impacts of SARS and pandemic influenza. In J. Duffin & A. Sweetman (eds), *SARS in Context: Memory, History, Policy.* Montreal: McGill-Queen's University Press, pp. 175–96.

Jernigan, D., Ragunathan, P., Bell, B., Brechner, R., Breznitz, E., Butler, J. et al. (2002). Investigation of bioterrorism-related anthrax, United States, 2001: Epidemiological findings. *Emerging Infectious Diseases,* 8, 1019–28.

Jodelet, D. (1991). *Madness and Social Representations.* Hertfordshire: Harvester and Wheatsheaf.

Joffe, H. (1999). *Risk and 'the Other'.* Cambridge: Cambridge University Press.

Joffe, H. & Haarhoff, G. (2002). Representations of far-flung illnesses: The case of Ebola in Britain. *Social Science & Medicine,* 54, 955–69.

Joffe, H. & Lee, N. (2004). Social representation of a food risk: The Hong Kong avian bird flu epidemic. *Journal of Health Psychology,* 9, 517–33.

Johnson, P. & Mueller, J. (2002). Updating the Accounts: Global Mortality of the 1918–1920 'Spanish' Influenza Pandemic. *Bulletin of the History of Medicine,* 76, 105–15.

Johnson, R., Nahmias, A., Magder, L., Lee, F., Brooks, C., & Snowden, C. (1989). A seroepidemiologic survey of the prevalence of herpes simplex virus type 2 infection in the United States. *New England Journal of Medicine,* 321, 7–12.

Jones, E. (2004). *A Matron's Charter: An Action Plan for Cleaner Hospitals* Leeds: NHS Estates.

Jones, K., Patel, N., Levy, M., Storeygard, A., Balk, D., Gittleman, J. et al. (2008). Global trends in emerging infectious diseases. *Nature,* 451, 990–3.

Kadlec, R., Zellicoff, A., & Vrtis, A. (1999). Biological weapons control: Prospects and implications for the future. In J. Lederberg (ed.), *Biological Weapons: Limiting the Threat.* Cambridge, MA: The MIT Press, pp. 95–112.

Kanki, P., Alroy, J., & Essex, M. (1985). Isolation of T-lymphotrophic retrovirus related to HTLV-III/LAV in wild caught African green monkeys. *Science,* 230, 951–4.

Kaufmann, S. (2009). *The New Plagues: Pandemics and Poverty in a Globalized World.* London: Haus Publishing.

Khardori, N. (2002). Vancomycin-resistant Enterococci. In F. Lashley & J. Durham (eds), *Emerging Infectious Diseases: Trends and Issues*. New York: Springer Publishing Company, pp. 243–54.

King, E. (1993). *Safety in Numbers*. London & New York: Cassell.

King, N. (2002). Security, disease, commerce: Ideologies of postcolonial global health. *Social Studies of Science*, 32, 763–89.

King, N. (2003a). Immigration, race and geographies of difference in the tuberculosis pandemic. In M. Gandy & A. Zumla (eds), *The Return of the White Plague: Global Poverty and the 'New' Tuberculosis*. London: Verso, pp. 39–54.

King, N. (2003b). The influence of anxiety: September 11, bioterrorism, and American public health. *Journal for the History of Medicine*, 58, 441.

King, N. (2004). The scale politics of emerging diseases. *Osiris*, 19, 76.

Kingston, W. (2000). Antibiotics, invention and innovation. *Research Policy*, 29, 679–710.

Kitler, M., Gavinio, P. & Lavanchy, D. (2002). Influenza and the work of the World Health Organization. *Vaccine*, 20, S5–S14.

Kitzinger, J. (1995). The face of AIDS. In *Representations of Health, Illness and Handicap*. Chur, Switzerland: Harwood Academic Publishers, pp. 49–66.

Kitzinger, J. & Reilly, J. (1997). The rise and fall of risk reporting: Media coverage of human genetics research, 'false memory syndrome' and 'mad cow disease'. *European Journal of Communication*, 12, 319–50.

Kolata, G. (1999). *Flu: The Story of the Great Influenza Pandemic of 1918 and the Search for the Virus that Caused it*. New York: Touchstone.

Kraut, A. (1994). *Silent Travellers: Germs, Genes, and the 'Immigrant Menace'*. New York: Basic Books.

Kuiken, T., Fouchier, R., Rimmelzwaan, G. & Osterhaus, A. (2003). Emerging viral infections in a rapidly changing world. *Current Opinion in Biotechnology*, 14, 641–6.

Lacey, R. (1994). *Mad Cow Disease: The History of BSE in Britain*. England: Gypsela Publications.

Lamey, B. & Malemeka, N. (1982). Aspects cliniques et epidemiologiques de la cryptococcose a Kinshasa. *Medecine Tropicale*, 42, 507–11.

Lane, H. & Fauci, A. (2001). Bioterrorism on the home front: A new challenge for American medicine. *Journal of the American Medical Association*, 286, 2595–7.

Lang, T. (1998). BSE and CJD: Recent developments. In S. Razan (ed.), *The Mad Cow Crisis: Health and the Public Good*. London: UCL Press, pp. 65–85.

Larson, B., Nerlich, B., & Wallis, P. (2005). Metaphors and biorisks: The war on infectious diseases and invasive species. *Science Communication*, 26, 243–68.

Lashley, F. (2002). Cyclospora cayetanensis: Arriving via Guatemalan raspberries. In F. Lashley & J. Durham (eds), *Emerging Infectious Diseases: Trends and Issues*. New York: Springer Publishing Company, pp. 93–102.

Laurance, J. (2003, April 6). Focus: Something in the food. *Independent on Sunday*.

Lawrence, J., Kearns, R., Park, J., Bryder, L. & Worth, H. (2008). Discourses of disease: Representations of tuberculosis within New Zealand newspapers 2002–2004. *Social Science and Medicine*, 66, 727–39.

Leach, J. (1998). Madness, metaphors and miscommunication: The rhetorical life of mad cow disease in Britain. In S. Razan (ed.), *The Mad Cow Crisis: Health and the Public Good*. London: UCL Press, pp. 119–30.

Lederberg, J. (1999). *Biological Weapons: Limiting the Threat.* Cambridge, MA: The MIT Press.

Lederberg, J., Shope, R., & Oaks, S. (1992). *Emerging Infections: Microbial Threats to Health in the United States.* Washington, DC: National Academy Press.

LeDuc, J., Childs, J., Glass, G. & Watson, A. (1993). Hantaan (Korean hemorrhagic fever) and related rodent zoonoses. In S.S. Morse (ed.), *Emerging Viruses.* New York and Oxford: Oxford University Press, pp. 149–58.

Lemert, C. (1987). *Postmodernism Is Not What You Think.* Oxford: Blackwell Publishers.

Levy, E. & Fischetti, M. (2003). *The New Killer Diseases: How the Alarming Evolution of Mutant Germs Threatens Us All.* New York: Crown Publishers.

Lewison, G. (2008). The reporting of the risks from severe acute respiratory syndrome (SARS) in the news media, 2003–2004. *Health, Risk and Society*, 10, 241–62.

Lewontin, R. & Levins, R. (2003). The return of old diseases and the appearance of new ones. In M. Gandy & A. Zumla (eds), *The Return of the White Plague: Global Poverty and the 'New' Tuberculosis.* London: Verso, pp. 1–6.

Livingstone, D. (1999). Tropical climate and moral hygiene: The anatomy of a Victorian debate. *British Journal for the History of Science*, 32, 93–110.

Lockerbie, S. & Herring, D. (2009). Global panic, local repercussions: Economic and nutritional effects of bird flu in Vietnam. In R. Hahn & M. Inhorn (eds), *Anthropology and Public Health.* Oxford: Oxford University Press, pp. 754–78.

Lupton, D. (1994). *Moral Threats and Dangerous Desires: AIDS in the News Media.* London: Taylor and Francis.

Lupton, D. (1999a). Archetypes of infection: People with HIV/AIDS in the Australian press in the mid 1990s. *Sociology of Health and Illness*, 21, 37–53.

Lupton, D. (1999b). *Risk.* London and New York: Routledge.

MacDougall, H. (2006). From Cholera to SARS: Communicable disease control procedures in Toronto 1832 to 2003. In J. Duffin & A. Sweetman (eds), *SARS in Context: Memory, History, Policy.* Montreal: McGill-Queen's University Press, pp. 79–104.

Martin, E. (1994). *Flexible Bodies: Tracking Immunity in American Culture from the Days of Polio to the Age of AIDS.* Boston: Beacon Press.

Mass, L. (2004). Hepatitis C and the news media: Lessons from AIDS. In R. Packard, P. Brown, R. Berkelman & H. Frumkin (eds), *Emerging Illness and Society: Negotiating the Public Health Agenda.* Baltimore and London: The Johns Hopkins University Press, pp. 388–405.

Masters, W., Johnson, V., & Kolodny, R. (1988). *Crisis: Heterosexual Behaviour in the Age of AIDS.* London: Weidenfeld and Nicolson.

Matricardi, P., Rosmini, F., Riondino, S., Fortini, M., Ferrigno, L., Rapicetta, M. et al. (2000). Exposure to foodborne and orofecal microbes versus airborne viruses in relation to atopy and allergic asthma: Epidemiological study. *British Medical Journal*, 320, 412–17.

Matsumoto, G. (2003). Anthrax powder: State of the art? *Science*, 302, 1492.

May, T. (2005). Funding agendas: Has bioterror defense been over-prioritized? *The American Journal of Bioethics*, 5, 34–44.

McKeown, T. (1976). *The Modern Rise of Population.* London: Edward Arnold.

Miller, D. (1999). Risk, science and policy: Definitional struggles, information management, the media and BSE. *Social Science and Medicine*, 49, 1239–55.

Miller, J., Engelberg, S., & Broad, W. (2001). *Germs: Biological Weapons and America's Secret War*. New York: Simon & Schuster.

Moeller, S. (1999). *Compassion Fatigue: How the Media sell Disease, Famine, War and Death*. New York and London: Routledge.

Moore, P., Harrison, L., Telzac, G., Ajello, G., & Broome, C. (1988). Group A meningococcal carriage in travelers returning from Saudi Arabia. *Journal of the American Medical Association*, 260, 2686–9.

Moreno, J. (2003). Introduction. In J. Moreno (ed.), *In the Wake of Terror: Medicine and Morality in a Time of Crisis*. Cambridge, MA: The MIT Press, pp. xv–xxxv.

Morse, S.S. (1992a). Examining the origins of emerging viruses. In S.S. Morse (ed.), *Emerging Viruses*. Oxford: Oxford University Press, pp. 10–28.

Morse, S.S. (1992b). Preface. In S.S. Morse (ed.), *Emerging Viruses*. Oxford: Oxford University Press, pp. i.

Morse, S.S. (1995). Factors in the emergence of infectious diseases. *Emerging Infectious Diseases*, 1, 7–15.

Moulin, A. (2000). The defended body. In R. Cooter & J. Pickstone (eds), *Medicine in the Twentieth Century*. Amsterdam: Harwood Academic, pp. 385–98.

Muraskin, W. (1993). Hepatitis B as a model (and anti-model) for AIDS. In V. Berridge & P. Strong (eds), *AIDS and Contemporary History*. Cambridge: Cambridge University Press, pp. 108–34.

Myers, G., MacInnes, K. & Myers, L. (1992). Phylogenetic moments in the AIDS epidemic. In S.S. Morse (ed.), *Emerging Viruses*. New York and Oxford: Oxford University Press, pp. 120–37.

National Intelligence Council (2000). *The Global Infectious Disease Threat and its Implications for the United States* Washington, DC: CIA.

National Science and Technology Council (1995). *Global Microbial Threats in the 1990s: Report of the NSTC Committee on International Science, Engineering and Technology (CISET) Working Group on Emerging and Re-emerging Infectious Diseases*. Washington, DC: CISET.

Nelkin, D. & Gilman, S. (1988). Placing blame for devastating disease. *Social Research*, 55, 361–78.

Nerlich, B. & Koteyko, N. (2008). Balancing food risks and food benefits: The coverage of probiotics in the UK national press. *Sociological Research Online*, 13, 1–16.

O'Conner, E. (2000). *Raw Material: Producing Pathology in Victorian Culture*. Durham and London: Duke University Press.

O'Toole, T. & Inglesby, T. (2003). Toward biosecurity. *Biosecurity and Bioterrorism: Biodefense Strategy, Practice and Science*, 1, 1.

O'Toole, T., Mair, M., & Inglesby, T. (2002). Shining light on 'Dark Winter'. *Clinical Infectious Diseases*, 34, 972–83.

Oldstone, M. (1998). *Viruses, Plagues and History*. Oxford: Oxford University Press.

Oleske, J., Minnefor, A., Cooper, R., Thomas, K., Cruz, A., Ahdieh, H. et al. (1983). Immune deficiency syndrome in children. *Journal of the American Medical Association*, 249, 2345–9.

Olson, K. (1999). Aum Shinrikyo: Once and future threat? *Emerging Infectious Diseases*, 5, 513–16.

Omran, A. (1971). The epidemiological transition: A theory of the epidemiology of population change. *Millbank Memorial Fund Quarterly*, 49, 509–38.

Omran, A. (1983). The epidemiological transition theory: A preliminary update. *Journal of Tropical Pediatrics*, 29, 305–16.

Oxford, J. (2001). The so-called great Spanish influenza pandemic of 1918 may have originated in France in 1916. *Philosophical Transactions of the Royal Society of London Series B*, 356, 1857–9.

Packard, R. (1989). *White Plague, Black Labor: Tuberculosis and the Political Economy of Health and Disease in South Africa*. Berkeley and Los Angeles: University of California Press.

Palumbi, S. (2001a). Humans as the world's greatest evolutionary force. *Science*, 293, 1786–90.

Palumbi, S. (2001b). *The Evolution Explosion: How Humans Can Cause Rapid Evolutionary Change*. New York: WW Norton and Co.

Park, K. (1993). Kimberley Bergalis, AIDS and the plague metaphor. In M. Garber, J. Matlock, & R. Walkowitz (eds), *Media Spectacles*. New York and London: Routledge, pp. 232–54.

Peden, A., Head, M., Richie, D., Bell, J. & Ironside, J. (2004). Preclinical vCJD after blood transfusion in a PRNP codon 129 heterozygous patient. *The Lancet*, 364, 527–9.

Pennington, T.H. (2003). *When Food Kills: BSE, E. Coli and Disaster Science*. Oxford: Oxford University Press.

Pernick, M. (2002). Contagion and culture. *American Literary History*, 14, 858–65.

Peters, C., Johnson, E., Jahrling, P., Ksiazek, T., Rollin, P., White, J. et al. (1993). Filoviruses. In S.S. Morse (ed.), *Emerging Viruses*. Oxford: Oxford University Press, pp. 159–75.

Pettifor, A. (2006). *The Coming First World Debt Crisis*. Basingstoke: Palgrave Macmillan.

Phillips, D. (1994). Epidemiological transition: Implications for health and health care provision. *Geografiska Annaler Series B, Human Geography*, 76, 71–89.

Piller, C. & Yamamoto, K. (1988). *Gene Wars: Military Control Over the New Genetic Technologies*. New York: Beech Tree Books.

Pisani, E. (2008). *The Wisdom of Whores: Bureaucrats, Brothels, and the Business of AIDS*. London: Grant Books.

Poirier, R. (1988). AIDS and traditions of homophobia. *Social Research*, 55, 461–75.

Poltorak, M., Leach, M., Fairhead, J., & Cassell, J. (2005). 'MMR talk' and vaccination choices: An ethnographic study in Brighton. *Social Science and Medicine*, 61, 709–19.

Preston, R. (1995). *The Hot Zone: A Terrifying True Story*. New York: Knopf Doubleday.

Preston, R. (1997). *The Cobra Event*. Toronto and New York: Random House.

Proctor, R. (1995). *Cancer Wars: How Politics Shapes What We Know and Don't Know About Cancer*. New York: Basic Books.

Read, T., Salzberg, S., Pop, M., Shumway, M., Umayam, L., Jiang, L. et al. (2002). Comparative genome sequencing for discovery of novel polymorphisms in Bacillus anthracis. *Science*, 296, 2028–33.

Reichman, L. & Tanne, J. (2002). *Timebomb: The Global Epidemic of Multi drug Resistant Tuberculosis*. New York: McGraw Hill.

Renne, E. (2006). Perspectives on polio and immunization in northern Nigeria. *Social Science and Medicine*, 63, 1857–69.

Rice, L. (2001). Emergence of vancomycin-resistant enterococci. *Emerging Infectious Diseases*, 7, 183–7.

Roberts, C. & Cox, M. (2003). *Health and Disease in Britain: From Prehistory to the Present Day*. Stroud: Sutton Publishing.

Rook, A. & Stanford, J. (1998). Give us this day our daily germs. *Immunology Today*, 19, 113–16.

Rosenberg, BH (2002, 22 September). Anthrax attacks push open an ominous door. *Los Angeles Times*.

Ryan, F. (1992). *The Forgotten Plague: How the Battle Against Tuberculosis Was Won – and Lost*. Boston, Toronto and London: Little Brown and Company.

Sabatier, R. (1988). *Blaming Others: Prejudice, Race and Worldwide AIDS*. London: Panos Publications Ltd.

Sachs, J. (2007). *Good Germs, Bad Germs: Health and Survival in a Bacterial World*. New York: Hill and Wang.

Said, E. (1978). *Orientalism*. London: Penguin Books.

Salkin, A (2006, 11 May). Germs never sleep. *The New York Times*.

Sarasin, P. (2006). *Anthrax: Bioterror as Fact and Fantasy*. Cambridge, MA: Harvard University Press.

Schaub, B., Lauener, R., & von Mutius, E. (2006). The many faces of the hygiene hypothesis. *The Journal of Allergy and Clinical Immunology*, 117, 969–77.

Schiller, N., Crystal, S., & Lewellen, D. (1994). Risky business: The cultural construction of AIDS risk groups. *Social Science & Medicine*, 38, 1337–46.

Scholten, B. (2007). Dirty Cows: Perceptions of BSE/vCJD. In B. Campkin & R. Cox (eds), *Dirt: New Geographies of Cleanliness and Contamination*. London and New York: IB Tauris, pp. 189–97.

Schwartz, B. & Yogev, R. (1996). An epidemic of emerging infectious diseases? *Seminars in Pediatric Infectious Diseases*, 7, 226–30.

Scott, C. (1896). Old age and death. *American Journal of Psychology*, 8, 67–122.

Shapiro, R. (2008). *Suckers: How Alternative Medicine Makes Fools of Us All*. London: Harvill Secker.

Shears, P. (2007). Poverty and infection in the developing world: Healthcare-related infections and infection control in the tropics. *Journal of Hospital Infection*, 67, 217–24.

Shell, R. (2000). Halfway to the holocaust: The economic, demographic and social implications of the AIDS pandemic to the year 2010 in the Southern African region. In *HIV/AIDS: A Threat to the African Renaissance? Konrad-Adenauer-Stiftung Occasional Papers*, June.

Shilts, R. (1987). *And the Band Played On: Politics, People and the AIDS Epidemic*. New York: Penguin Books.

Shnayerson, M. & Plotkin, M. (2002). *The Killers Within: The Deadly Rise of Drug Resistant Bacteria*. Boston, New York and London: Little Brown and Company.

Shohat, E. & Stam, R. (1994). *Unthinking Eurocentrism: Multiculturalism and the Media*. London: Routledge.

Shove, E. (2003). *Comfort, Cleanliness and Convenience: The Social Organization of Normality*. Oxford: Berg.

Showalter, E. (1997). *Hystories: Hysterical Epidemics and Modern Media*. New York: Columbia University Press.

Sidel, V., Hillel, W., & Gould, R. (2001). Good intentions and the road to bioterrorism preparedness. *American Journal of Public Health*, 91, 716–17.

Singel, L. & Lashley, F. (2009). Cholera. In F. Lashley & J. Durham (eds), *Emerging Infectious Diseases: Trends and Issues*. New York: Springer Publishing Company, pp. 73–82.

Singer, M. & Clair, S. (2003). Syndemics and public health: Reconceptualizing disease in a bio-social context. *Medical Anthropology Quarterly*, 17, 423–41.

Singh, J., Hallmayer, J., & Illes, J. (2007). Interacting and paradoxical forces in neuroscience and society. *Nature Reviews Neuroscience*, 8, 153–60.

Smallman-Raynor, M. & Cliff, A. (2003). War and disease: Some perspectives on the spatial and temporal occurence of tuberculosis in wartime. In M. Gandy & A. Zumla (eds), *The Return of the White Plague: Global Poverty and the 'New' Tuberculosis*. London: Verso, pp. 70–94.

Smith, P. (2001). *Cultural Theory: An Introduction*. Malden, MA: Blackwell Publishers.

Smith, V. (2007). *Clean: A History of Personal Hygiene and Purity*. Oxford: Oxford University Press.

Smith-Nonini, S. (2004). The cultural politics of institutional responses to resurgent tuberculosis epidemics: New York City and Lima, Peru. In R. Packard, P. Brown, R. Berkelman, & H. Frumkin (eds), *Emerging Illness and Society: Negotiating the Public Health Agenda*. Baltimore and London: The Johns Hopkins University Press, pp. 253–90.

Sontag, S. (1978). *Illness as Metaphor*. London: Penguin Books.

Sontag, S. (1989). *AIDS and its metaphors*. (Penguin Books 1991 ed.) USA: Farrar, Straus & Giroux.

Spier, R. (2002). Perception of risk of vaccine adverse events: A historical perspective. *Vaccine*, 20, S78–S84.

Spurgeon, D. (2007). Prevalence of MRSA in US hospitals hits a new high. *British Medical Journal*, 335, 961.

Stanford, J. & Grange, J. (1991). Is Africa lost? *The Lancet*, 338, 557–9.

Stern, J. (1999). *The Ultimate Terrorists*. Cambridge, MA: Harvard University Press.

Stern, V. (2003). *The House of the Dead* revisited: Prisons, tuberculosis and public health in the former Soviet bloc. In M. Gandy & A. Zumla (eds), *The Return of the White Plague: Global Poverty and the 'New' Tuberculosis*. London: Verso, pp. 178–94.

Stetten, D. (1980). Eradication. *Science*, 210, 1203.

Stokes, G. (2002). Microbial resistance to antibiotics. In F. Lashley & J. Durham (eds), *Emerging Infectious Diseases: Trends and Issues*. New York: Springer Publishing Company, pp. 23–42.

Strachan, D. (1989). Hay fever, hygiene, and household size. *British Medical Journal*, 299, 1259–60.

Streefland, P., Chowdhury, A., & Ramos-Jimenez, P. (1999). Patterns of vaccination acceptance. *Social Science and Medicine*, 49, 1705–16.

Strong, P. (1990). Epidemic psychology: A model. *Sociology of Health and Illness*, 12, 249–59.

Tartasky, D. (2002). Escherichia coli O157:H7. In F. Lashley & J. Durham (eds), *Emerging Infectious Diseases: Trends and Issues*. New York: Springer Publishing Company, pp. 129–38.

Taubenberger, J., Reid A.H., Janczewski A. & Fanning T.G. (2001). Integrating historical, clinical and molecular genetic data in order to explain the origin and virulence of the 1918 Spanish influenza virus. *Philosophical Transactions of the Royal Society of London Series B*, 356, 1829–39.

Tauxe, R. (1997). Emerging foodborne diseases: An evolving public health challenge. *Emerging Infectious Diseases*, 3, 425–34.

Taylor, L., Latham, S., & Woolhouse, E. (2001). Risk factors for human disease emergence. *Philosophical Transactions of the Royal Society of London*, 356, 983–9.

The BSE Inquiry (2000). *Report, Evidence and Supporting Papers of the Inquiry into the Emergence and Identification of Bovine Spongiform Encephalopathy (BSE) and Variant Creutzfeldt-Jakob Disease (vCJD) and the Action Taken in Response to it up to 20 March 1996*. London: HMSO.

The National Creutzfeldt-Jakob Disease Surveillance Unit (2009). vCJD worldwide. The University of Edinburgh (On-line). Available: http://www.cjd.ed.ac.uk/.

Tiffin, H. (2007). Foot in Mouth: Animals, disease and the cannibal complex. *Mosaic*, 40, 11–16.

Tognotti, E. (2003). Scientific triumphalism and learning from the facts: Bacteriology and the 'Spanish flu' challenge of 1918. *The Journal of the Society for the Social History of Medicine*, 16, 97–110.

Treichler, P. (1999). *How to Have Theory in an Epidemic: Cultural Chronicles of AIDS*. Durham, NC: Duke University Press.

Treichler, P. (1988). AIDS gender and biomedical discourse: Current contests for meaning. In E. Fee & D. Fox (eds), *AIDS: The Burdens of History*. Berkeley: University of California Press, pp. 190–266.

Trotter, G. (2003). Emergency medicine, terrorism, and universal access to health care: A potent mixture for erstwhile knights-errant. In J. Moreno (ed.), *In the Wake of Terror: Medicine and Morality in a Time of Terror*. Cambridge, MA: The MIT Press, pp. 133–47.

Trust for America's Health (2006). Covering the pandemic flu threat: Tracking atricles and some key events, 1997 to 2005. Trust for American's Health (On-line). Available: http://healthyamericans.org/reports/flumedia/Covering Report.pdf.

Ungar, S. (1998). Hot crises and media reassurance: A comparison of emerging diseases and Ebola Zaire. *British Journal of Sociology*, 49, 36–56.

Urquhart, J. & Heilmann, K. (1984). *Risk Watch; The Odds of Life*. New York: Facts on File Publications.

Victor, T. & Young, D. (2005). Tackling the white plague: Multidrug-resistant tuberculosis. In G. Newton (ed.), *Antibiotic Resistance: An Unwinnable War*. London: The Wellcome Trust, pp. 29–31.

Vigarello, G. (1988). *Concepts of Cleanliness: Changing Attitudes in France Since the Middle Ages*. Cambridge: Cambridge University Press.

Wakefield, A., Murch, S., Anthony, A., Linnell, J., Casson, D., Malik, M. et al. (1998). Ileal-lymphoid-nodular hyperplasia, non-specific colitis, and pervasive developmental disorder in children. *The Lancet*, 351, 637–41.

Wallace, D. & Wallace, R. (1998). *A Plague on Your Houses: How New York was Burned Down and Public Health Crumbled*. London and New York: Verso.

Wallace, D. & Wallace, R. (2003). The recent tuberculosis epidemic in New York City: Warning from the de-developing world. In M. Gandy & A. Zumla (eds), *The Return of the White Plague: Global Poverty and the 'New' Tuberculosis*. London: Verso, pp. 125–46.

Wallis, P. & Nerlich, B. (2005). Disease metaphors in new epidemics: The UK media framing of the 2003 SARS epidemic. *Social Science & Medicine*, 60, 2629–39.

Washer, P. (2004). Representations of SARS in the British newspapers. *Social Science & Medicine*, 59, 2561–71.

Washer, P. (2006). Representations of mad cow disease. *Social Science & Medicine*, 62, 457–66.

Washer, P. & Joffe, H. (2006). The 'hospital superbug': Social representations of MRSA. *Social Science & Medicine*, 63, 2141–52.

Washer, P., Joffe, H., & Solberg, C. (2008). Audience readings of media messages about MRSA. *Journal of Hospital Infection*, 70, 42–7.

Watney, S. (1987). *Policing Desire: Pornography, AIDS and the Media*. London: Cassell.

Watney, S. (1989). Taking liberties. In E. Carter & S. Watney (eds), *Taking Liberties: AIDS and Cultural Politics*. London: Serpents Tail, pp. 11–58.

Watney, S. (1994). *Practices of Freedom: Selected Writings on HIV/AIDS*. London: Rivers Oram Press.

Weeks, J. (1993). AIDS and the regulation of sexuality. In V. Berridge & P. Strong (eds), *AIDS and Contemporary History*. Cambridge: Cambridge University Press, pp. 17–36.

Weinberg, J. & Simmonds, S. (1995). Public health, epidemiology and war. *Social Science and Medicine*, 40, 1663–9.

Weir, S. & Beetham, D. (1998). *What the Public Give: Political Power and Accountability in British Government*. London: Routledge.

Weisman, S.R (2005, 9 November). Powell calls his UN speech a lasting blot on his record. *The New York Times*.

Weiss, R. & McMichael, A. (2004). Social and environmental risk factors in the emergence of infectious diseases. *Nature Medicine*, 10, 1150.

Wellcome Witnesses to Twentieth Century Medicine (2000). *Post Penicillin Antibiotics: From Acceptance to Resistance* London: The Wellcome Institute.

Welshman, J. (2000). Tuberculosis and ethnicity in England and Wales, 1950–70. *Sociology of Health and Illness*, 22, 858–82.

Wetter, D., Daniell, W., & Treser, C. (2001). Hospital preparedness for victims of chemical or biological terrorism. *American Journal of Public Health*, 91, 710–16.

Widdus, R. (1999). The potential to control or eradicate infectious diseases through immunisation. *Vaccine*, 17, S6–S12.

Wilkinson, I. (2001). Social theories of risk perception: At once indispensable and insufficient. *Current Sociology*, 49, 1–22.

Williamson, J. (1989). Every virus tells a story: The meanings of HIV and AIDS. In E. Carter & S. Watney (eds), *Taking Liberties: AIDS and Cultural Politics*. London: Serpent's Tail, pp. 69–80.

Wilson, M. (1995). Travel and the emergence of infectious diseases. *Emerging Infectious Diseases*, 1, 39–46.

Winslow, C. (1943). *The Conquest of Epidemic Disease: A Chapter in the History of Ideas*. Wisconsin: University of Wisconsin Press.

Wolfe, R. & Sharp, L. (2002). Anti-vaccinationists past and present. *British Medical Journal*, 325, 430–2.

World Health Organization (1978). *Declaration of Alma-Ata: International Conference on Primary Health Care, Alma-Ata, USSR, 6–12 September 1978* Geneva: World Health Organization.

World Health Organization (2003a). *Cumulative Number of Reported Probable Cases of SARS from 1 Nov 2002 to 11 July 2003* Geneva: World Health Organization.

World Health Organization (2003b). *Dr. Carlo Urbani of the World Health Organization Dies of SARS* Geneva: World Health Organization.

World Health Organization (2003c). *Severe Acute Respiratory Syndrome (SARS): Resolution of the 56th World Health Assembly* (Rep. No. WHA56.29). Geneva: World Health Organization.

World Health Organization (2009). *Confirmed Human Cases of Avian Influenza A (H5N1)* Geneva: World Health Organization.

Wynia, M. (2006). Risk and trust in public health: A cautionary tale. *The American Journal of Bioethics*, 6, 3–6.

Zambon, M. & Nicholson, KG. (2003). Sudden acute respiratory syndrome. *British Medical Journal*, 326, 669.

Zinsser, H. (1935). *Rats, Lice and History*. London: George Routledge and Sons Ltd.

Index